NEW DIRECTIONS FOR PROGRAM EVAL
A Publication of the American Evaluation Association

Nick L. Smith, *Syracuse University*
EDITOR-IN-CHIEF

Evaluating AIDS Prevention: Contributions of Multiple Disciplines

Laura C. Leviton
University of Pittsburgh

Andrea M. Hegedus
University of Pittsburgh

Alan Kubrin
University of Pittsburgh

EDITORS

Number 46, Summer 1990

JOSSEY-BASS INC., PUBLISHERS
San Francisco • Oxford

Evaluating AIDS Prevention: Contributions of Multiple Disciplines.
Laura C. Leviton, Andrea M. Hegedus, Alan Kubrin (eds.).
New Directions for Program Evaluation, no. 46.

NEW DIRECTIONS FOR PROGRAM EVALUATION
Nick L. Smith, Editor-in-Chief

Copyright © 1990 by Jossey-Bass Inc., Publishers

Copyright under International, Pan American, and Universal
Copyright Conventions. All rights reserved. No part of
this issue may be reproduced in any form—except for a brief
quotation (not to exceed 500 words) in a review or professional
work—without permission in writing from the publishers.

NEW DIRECTIONS FOR PROGRAM EVALUATION is part of The Jossey-Bass
Higher Education and Social and Behavioral Science Series and is published
quarterly by Jossey-Bass Inc., Publishers (publication number USPS 449-050).

EDITORIAL CORRESPONDENCE should be sent to the Editor-in-Chief,
Nick L. Smith, School of Education, Syracuse University,
330 Huntington Hall, Syracuse, New York 13244-2340.

Library of Congress Catalog Card Number LC 85-644749
International Standard Serial Number ISSN 0164-7989
International Standard Book Number ISBN 1-55542-835-5

Manufactured in the United States of America. Printed on acid-free paper.

NEW DIRECTIONS FOR PROGRAM EVALUATION
Sponsored by the American Evaluation Association
(A Joint Organization of the Evaluation Research Society and the Evaluation Network)

EDITOR-IN-CHIEF
Nick L. Smith   Education, Syracuse University

EDITORIAL ASSISTANT
Eileen E. Schroeder   Education, Syracuse University

EDITORIAL ADVISORY BOARD

Gerald L. Barkdoll   U.S. Food and Drug Administration, Washington, D.C.
Leonard B. Bickman   Program Evaluation Laboratory, Vanderbilt University
Robert F. Boruch   Psychology and Statistics, Northwestern University
Donald T. Campbell   Social Relations, Lehigh University
Thomas D. Cook   Psychology, Northwestern University
David S. Cordray   U.S. General Accounting Office, Washington, D.C.
David M. Fetterman   School of Education, Stanford University
Barry J. Fraser   Curtin University, Western Australia
Jennifer C. Greene   Human Service Studies, Cornell University
Edward H. Haertel   School of Education, Stanford University
Ernest R. House   School of Education, University of Colorado, Boulder
Michael H. Kean   CTB-McGraw-Hill, Monterey, California
Morris Lai   College of Education, University of Hawaii
Laura C. Leviton   Health Services Administration, University of Pittsburgh
Richard J. Light   Education, Harvard University
Mark W. Lipsey   Psychology, Claremont Graduate School
Jennifer McCreadie   Madison Metropolitan School District (Wisconsin)
Jack McKillip   Psychology, Southern Illinois University, Carbondale
Anna Madison   Public Affairs, Texas Southern University
Jeanne C. Marsh   School of Social Service Administration,
                               University of Chicago
Carol T. Mowbray   Resident and Evaluation Division, Michigan Department
                               of Mental Health
David Nevo   Education, Tel Aviv University
Dianna L. Newman   Evaluation Consortium, SUNY-Albany
Dennis Palumbo   School of Justice Studies, Arizona State University
Michael Q. Patton   Minnesota Extension Service, University of Minnesota
Mark St. John   Inverness Research Associates, Inverness, California
Thomas A. Schwandt   Educational Psychology, Northern Illinois University
Lee B. Sechrest   Psychology, University of Arizona
William R. Shadish, Jr.   Psychology, Memphis State University
John K. Smith   Education, University of Northern Iowa
Charles B. Stalford   OERI, Washington, D.C.
Carol H. Weiss   Education, Harvard University

AMERICAN EVALUATION ASSOCIATION, 9555 PERSIMMON TREE ROAD, POTOMAC, MD 20854

Contents

EDITORS' NOTES 1
Laura C. Leviton, Andrea M. Hegedus, Alan Kubrin

1. AIDS Prevention: A Public Health Psychology Perspective 7
Deborah L. Rugg
No single, one-shot intervention will adequately influence AIDS prevention. Rather, a sustained, multidimensional effort with repeated exposures to a variety of well-planned and targeted strategies is essential.

2. An Overview of AIDS Modeling 23
Edward H. Kaplan
Mathematical models of the AIDS epidemic have been used in forecasts, scientific estimations of disease parameters, and policy analyses. The author reviews several modeling approaches and their uses, stressing results most relevant to policy analysts and program evaluators.

3. Estimates of AIDS Incubation Periods from Convenience Samples 37
Paul R. Abramson, Richard A. Berk
The authors question current estimates of the AIDS incubation period drawn from convenience samples, citing potential difficulties with generalizability and selection bias.

4. Ethnographic Evaluation of AIDS Prevention Programs: Better Data for Better Programs 51
Jean J. Schensul, Stephen L. Schensul
Ethnographic methods provide contextual and culturally sensitive information to AIDS administrators and service providers. This chapter discusses current informational needs in AIDS prevention programs, examines the interplay of ethnology and evaluation, and describes the steps in ethnographic evaluation.

5. A Model for AIDS Education 63
Douglas Longshore
This chapter reviews the model developed by the General Accounting Office for AIDS education, compares it to models in other public health campaigns, and suggests seven factors that should be considered in any AIDS prevention campaign.

6. Theory-Based Evaluation of AIDS-Related Knowledge, Attitudes, and 75
Behavior Changes
Ross F. Conner, Shiraz I. Mishra, Megan A. Lewis, Samantha Bryer, Jeff Marks, Mini Lai, Lisa Clark
Three theoretical approaches to disease prevention and health promotion are discussed in this chapter. The authors then present an example of an AIDS prevention program that used these theories to formulate the intervention and to guide the evaluation research.

7. AIDS Prevention Programs: The Need for Evaluation in the Context 87
of Community Partnership
Joanne E. Mantell, Anthony T. DiVittis
The authors examine strategies for developing, implementing, and evaluating effective AIDS prevention programs. These strategies are presented in the context of a partnership between the evaluator and the target community.

NAME INDEX 99

SUBJECT INDEX 105

Editors' Notes

By any criteria, AIDS presents one of the most serious challenges to our society today. Whereas the first 50,000 AIDS cases were reported to the Centers for Disease Control (CDC) during six years, from 1981 to 1987, the second 50,000 cases were reported within only a year and a half, between December 1987 and July 1989. Close to 60 percent of the cases have been fatal (Centers for Disease Control, 1989b). Although projections vary, 330,000 cases are predicted in the U.S. by 1992 (Centers for Disease Control, 1989a). Access to medical care for people with AIDS and the cost of that care both to the individual and to society present formidable problems (National Organizations Responding to AIDS, 1988; Pascal, 1987).

The prevention of AIDS through such methods as health education, social marketing, and community organization remains the only tool at hand for containing the epidemic, much less ending it. Social scientists have been involved in studies of AIDS prevention for some time. Psychologists, public health and medical professionals, social workers, anthropologists, and others have all adapted their frameworks and experience to tailor interventions for individuals and groups that engage in high-risk behaviors. However, most of the professionals involved would agree that the evaluation of these interventions is an important component of AIDS prevention that needs considerable improvement. This sourcebook provides frameworks from several disciplines for overall improvement in the evaluation of AIDS prevention.

The quality of evaluation for AIDS prevention has lagged behind that of intervention for several reasons. The most important reasons have been the lack of leadership and funding on both the federal and the state levels. Many view the federal funding record as a true scandal (Shilts, 1987). Only in 1989 did federal funding for AIDS reach the level devoted to such other major diseases as cancer and heart disease. It is also the case that because of the stigma attached to the disease and to the groups who contract the disease, relatively few researchers were willing to become involved in the early years (Shilts, 1987). In the absence of governmental and research leadership, community organizations took the lead in prevention. Appropriately, they tended to assign priority for limited resources to intervention, any intervention, in the face of an epidemic that was overwhelming certain communities. As Joanne Mantell and Anthony DiVittis point out in Chapter Seven of this sourcebook, however, the absence of evidence on effectiveness has led some experts to question the existing prevention strategies and to offer less palatable alternatives. This experience has forced a move toward more rigorous evaluation. In this respect, the evaluation of AIDS prevention has followed the same course as evaluation in many other policy sectors (Cook, Leviton, and Shadish, 1985; Rossi and Freeman, 1989).

Improvements are needed both in the methods used to discover appropriate interventions and in the rigorous testing of the effectiveness of those interventions. Discovery of appropriate interventions entails improving the understanding of the ecology of high-risk behaviors, finding the means to access individuals and groups at high risk, seeking ways to influence the norms of the social networks involved, and developing communications and skills training to produce long-term maintenance of behavior changes. In the rigorous evaluation of the effectiveness of interventions we are faced with a host of challenges. The litany of problems includes but is not limited to choosing appropriate criteria for behavior change, validating behavior change, selecting samples that can be generalized to communities at risk or to the general population, maintaining longitudinal studies and preventing attrition, and converting any obtained behavior-change information into concrete expectations about effects, if any, on the epidemic.

Compounding these problems is the relative lack of prior information concerning groups that tend to engage in high-risk behavior. Not enough is known about sexual behavior in general, let alone the behavior of men who have sex with men. The ecology of needle sharing and of injection drug use is not well enough understood. Little is known about the sexual partners of injection drug users (Bell, 1989; Mondanaro, 1987). Furthermore, the epidemic is changing and the nature of drug use is changing with the creation of new risk factors for HIV infection in the "sex-for-crack" problem (Brown, 1989). In order to make policy decisions about prevention as a strategy, we also need more basic information about the epidemic itself. How many AIDS cases can we really expect? How much prevention is enough to stem the tide? How soon can this goal be accomplished?

Some progress is being made on all these fronts (Leviton and Valdiserri, 1990). While some techniques are being developed to begin to address these problems, they are already described in the AIDS prevention literature. What is missing from the literature is an explicit description of the range of theoretical frameworks, growing out of various disciplines, that have guided AIDS prevention research and evaluation. This volume aims at providing such descriptions.

Overview of Chapters

Comprehensive evaluation of AIDS prevention must borrow from several disciplines. AIDS has rapidly overwhelmed our traditional approaches to public health problems. Because of the broad range of problems it entails, narrow discipline-oriented approaches are grossly insufficient to combat AIDS. What is needed is a more multidimensional approach including, but not limited to, the knowledge bases of epidemiology, ethnography, behavioral theory, operations research, community organization studies, and model health education campaigns. Subsequently, this integrated approach must be rigorously evaluated at several levels in order to direct its growth and adapt it to the problems at hand. The initial step in such an approach is a description of the range of various theoretical and methodological options available to the evaluator.

In Chapter One, Deborah Rugg outlines a framework for the study of AIDS prevention that marries health psychology to the disciplines of epidemiology and public health practice. Priorities and criteria for evaluation are assigned in light of key concepts from this framework. The chapter is of great assistance in outlining the overlaps, in terms of concerns and questions asked, among these disciplines.

Chapters Two and Three focus on the ultimate goals of AIDS prevention programs. Just what is the course of this epidemic, anyway? How will behavior changes affect its course? How big would those changes have to be before we would say that prevention was successful? In Chapter Two, Edward Kaplan uses operations research methods to address those questions. Kaplan reviews mathematical models of the AIDS epidemic and shows how they can be used to inform policy analysis. One important implication of the AIDS models is that risk reduction at the level of populations does not have to be complete in order to stop the epidemic within a specified time period. This presentation is remarkable in that these models can set targets for risk reduction so that effect sizes for behavior change (that is, differences between groups on outcome measures) have concrete meaning. Such targets for effect size are rare in evaluation research (Yeaton and Sechrest, 1981).

In Chapter Three, Paul Abramson and Richard Berk show how experience derived from applied social sciences—and from evaluation in particular—contributes to AIDS epidemiology. The authors explain how convenience samples and censored samples adversely affect the validity of estimates of the time period from infection with the HIV virus to the contraction of AIDS. In doing so, they challenge important assumptions of epidemiology and illustrate problems in generalizing from such samples. The chapter is important to evaluation because without meaningful estimates of incubation, we cannot project confidently from intermediate outcomes, such as behaviors, to the ultimate variables of interest—the number of AIDS cases and their societal impact.

The next three chapters focus on the generation and testing of health behavior theory in AIDS program evaluation. In Chapter Four, Jean and Stephen Schensul make an excellent case for ethnography as a vital methodology for the evaluation of AIDS prevention programs. Indeed, we have seen few policy and program areas in which the case for using both qualitative and quantitative methods (in the sense that these authors advocate) is more persuasive than it is in AIDS prevention. The nature of the high-risk behaviors and their social contexts remain extremely difficult to study. Ethnographic methods have proved especially valuable in studying AIDS prevention demonstrations aimed at recruiting and educating injection drug users (IDUs) and their sexual partners. They have been shown to be important in validating self-reported behavior, in identifying social networks, and in identifying changes in the norms of those networks (Wiebel, 1988). Several of the principal investigators of demonstration projects for IDUs concluded at a recent meeting sponsored by the National Institute on Drug Abuse that evaluations of outcome are still premature. The scientific community still does not understand IDUs or their social context, and therefore the interventions cannot be as good as they need to be. Even the participants who advocated structured interviews acknowledged that measurement of individual behaviors in great detail has been stressed at the expense of understanding the social context.

In Chapter Five, Douglas Longshore presents a model of health education campaigns for AIDS prevention, developed by the Program Evaluation and Methodology Division of the U.S. General Accounting Office (GAO). The GAO surveyed AIDS prevention campaigns that were nominated as having exemplary characteristics, based on our current knowledge of health education. While the GAO did not formally evaluate the effectiveness of these campaigns, its survey is helpful to the evaluation community. Until more empirical evidence is available from AIDS prevention studies, the GAO model can guide the evaluator in selecting priorities for research questions.

In Chapter Six, Ross Conner and his colleagues apply three theories that have been specifically developed to predict and control individual health behavior change. These theories informed both the development and the evaluation of a university course on AIDS. The pre-experimental design examined change in knowledge, attitudes, and behavior related to AIDS risk. The focus on theory in evaluation is desirable, in our view. These theories are still evolving, however, and much remains to be discovered about the forces that influence behavior related to health. This lack is reflected in the literature, where studies employing such theories often do not capture much of the variance in intentions or actual behavior (Leventhal, Meyer, and Guttman, 1980).

Chapters One and Six reflect an ongoing debate that will influence the form taken by prevention and health education in the future. The theories applied by Conner and his colleagues assume essential causal relationships among knowledge, attitudes, and behavior. The model presented by Rugg assumes that under some circumstances the three constructs may not be directly related. Clearly, better AIDS prevention research can inform this debate, and evaluations of intermediate objectives need to consider more precisely the relationship of knowledge and attitudes to behavior change.

Community involvement continues to be a cornerstone of AIDS prevention activities (Freudenberg, Lee, and Silver, 1989). In Chapter Seven, Joanne Mantell and Anthony DiVittis illustrate the challenges and the opportunities provided by partnerships with target communities in evaluating AIDS prevention. They speak from experience—namely, their work with the Gay Men's Health Crisis of New York City and the New York City Department of Health. Their special version of the stakeholder evaluation offers opportunities for both formative and summative functions of evaluation.

Chapters Two and Seven highlight a dilemma for the valuing dimension of AIDS prevention evaluation. Affected communities may not have the same criteria for program success as the public health professional or policy maker. In many affected communities (where the prevalence of HIV infection is very high), individual risk still presents a life-or-death dilemma. Thus, we might find that these stakeholders advocate the absolute elimination of riskful behavior as the only acceptable criterion. Or they might set ambitious goals for the reduction of new infections within a specified time limit. In contrast, public health professionals and policy makers might find programs successful if they slowed the epidemic for populations as a whole. In these chapters, Kaplan's criteria for successful prevention are clearly based on populations as a whole, while Mantell and DiVittis look to both population and individual criteria for success. Our guess, however, is that all these authors would recognize the importance of both sets of criteria.

Conclusion

This sourcebook illustrates the conclusion that comprehensive evaluation generally borrows from multiple disciplines. Social work, anthropology, and public health practice focus on communities; health psychology and health education generally focus on individuals; epidemiology and many mathematical models focus on populations. The next step in the evolution of the evaluation of AIDS prevention programs is to begin integrating these approaches into a planned program of comprehensive evaluation.

The editors would like to acknowledge and thank the peer reviewers whose valuable critiques improved these manuscripts: Jacqueline Dunbar, Marigold Edwards, Herbert Schulberg, and Myrna Silverman of the University of Pittsburgh; William Shadish of Memphis State University; and Michael Dennis of Research Triangle Institute.

Laura C. Leviton
Andrea M. Hegedus
Alan Kubrin
Editors

References

Bell, N. K. "AIDS and Women: Remaining Ethical Issues." *AIDS Education and Prevention,* 1989, *1,* 22-30.

Brown, B. Keynote address presented to the first annual conference of National AIDS Demonstration Projects, Rockville, Md., October 16, 1989.

Centers for Disease Control. "AIDS and Human Immunodeficiency Virus Infection in the United States: 1988 Update." CDC Surveillance Supplements. *Morbidity and Mortality Weekly Report,* 1989a, *38* (S-4), entire issue.

Centers for Disease Control. "First 100,000 Cases of Acquired Immunodeficiency Syndrome—United States." *Morbidity and Mortality Weekly Report,* 1989b, *38,* 561–563.

Cook, T. D., Leviton, L. C., and Shadish, W. R. "Program Evaluation." In G. Lindsey and E. Aronson (eds.), *The Handbook of Social Psychology.* 3rd ed. New York: Random House, 1985.

Freudenberg, N., Lee, J., and Silver, D. "How Black and Latino Community Organizations Respond to the AIDS Epidemic: A Case Study in One New York City Neighborhood." *AIDS Education and Prevention,* 1989, *1,* 12-21.

Leventhal, H., Meyer, D., and Guttman, M. "The Role of Theory in the Study of Compliance to High Blood Pressure Regimens." In R. B. Haynes, M. E. Mattson, and O. E. Tillmer (eds.), *Patient Compliance to Prescribed Antihypertensive Medication Regimens: A Report to the National Heart, Lung, and Blood Institute.* Washington, D.C.: U.S. Department of Health and Human Services, 1980.

Leviton, L. C., and Valdiserri, R. O. "Evaluating AIDS Prevention: Outcome, Implementation, and Mediating Variables." *Evaluation and Program Planning,* 1990, *13* (1), 55-66.

Mondanaro, J. "Strategies for AIDS Prevention: Motivating Healthy Behavior in Drug-Dependent Women." *Journal of Psychoactive Drugs,* 1987, *19,* 143-149.

National Organizations Responding to AIDS. *A Call for Executive Action: Recommendations to the Transition Team.* Washington, D.C.: AIDS Action Council, 1988.

Pascal, A. *The Costs of Treating AIDS Under Medicaid: 1986-1991.* Santa Monica, Calif.: Rand Corporation, 1987.

Rossi, P. H., and Freeman, H. E. *Evaluation: A Systematic Approach.* (4th ed.) Newbury Park, Calif.: Sage, 1989.

Shilts, R. *And the Band Played On: Politics, People, and the AIDS Epidemic.* New York: Penguin, 1987.

Wiebel, W. W. "Combining Ethnographic and Epidemiologic Methods in Targeted AIDS Interventions: The Chicago Model." In R. J. Battles and R. W. Pickens (eds.), *Needle Sharing Among Intravenous Drug Abusers: National and International Perspectives.* National Institute on Drug Abuse Research Monograph no. 80. Rockville, Md.: U.S. Department of Health and Human Services, 1988.

Yeaton, W. H., and Sechrest, L. "Estimating Effect Size." In P. M. Wortman (ed.), *Methods for Evaluating Health Services.* Beverly Hills, Calif.: Sage, 1981.

Laura C. Leviton is associate professor of community health services at the Graduate School of Public Health of the University of Pittsburgh.

Andrea M. Hegedus is a research associate at the Graduate School of Public Health of the University of Pittsburgh.

Alan Kubrin is a doctoral student at the Graduate School of Public Health of the University of Pittsburgh.

To prevent HIV infection we must influence risky sexual and drug-using practices, some of the most basic yet complex of human behaviors. No single discipline or one-shot intervention is going to solve this problem; rather, a sustained, multidimensional, interdisciplinary effort with repeat exposures to a variety of well-planned and targeted strategies is essential.

AIDS Prevention: A Public Health Psychology Perspective

Deborah L. Rugg

In recent years, specific knowledge from psychological theory and research has been extended beyond the treatment of individuals and small groups to focus on communities in an effort to influence the health of the nation. To apply this knowledge, psychologists and other behavioral scientists, including program evaluators, are needed in public health agencies. This combination of behavioral science and public health principles creates an applied technology for health promotion and disease prevention that is useful in many areas of public health. One of these areas, the development and evaluation of effective AIDS prevention strategies, requires such interdisciplinary efforts. To create an effective interdisciplinary effort, we must start by understanding the contributions of each other's discipline. This chapter describes contributions to AIDS prevention from a public health psychology perspective.

The opportunity for psychologists to be critically involved in solving a major public health problem through basic science research, applied research and program evaluation, clinical services, and legislative activities has never been greater. With the advent of the AIDS epidemic, increasing numbers of psychologists have joined front-line efforts in disease prevention and epidemic control. Many more are needed. However, since past involvement of psychologists in infectious disease control has been limited, education on the potential contributions of psychology to efforts to control AIDS is necessary for psychologists as well as for public health professionals and program evaluators.

In this chapter, I will briefly define health psychology and public health psychology and summarize current contributions of psychologists to the AIDS prevention and control effort. I will then discuss key concepts in AIDS prevention from a public health psychologist's perspective and end with recommendations for a research agenda for the evaluation of AIDS prevention.

Definitions

Health psychology is the psychological discipline devoted to studying and enhancing the health and well-being of individuals. Originally defined by Stone, Cohen, Adler, and Associates (1979), it is the application of psychological theory, treatment, and research to the development, maintenance, and restoration of physical and mental well-being. It involves a comprehensive approach to the understanding of human health, viewing the individual as an integrated biopsychosocial system and incorporating principles from a number of psychological disciplines. Examples of topics studied by health psychologists include the relationship between psychological factors, such as stress and coping, and the development of illness; the role of social supports in health outcomes; risk-taking behaviors, such as smoking, overeating, drinking, and unprotected sex; analysis and improvement of doctor-patient communications and other health transactions; theories of behavior and the role of various cognitions, attitudes, beliefs, and skills in initiating and maintaining changes in risk-taking behaviors; and improving the health care system and the formulation of health policy.

Public health psychology is a new field (Rugg, Hovell, and Franzini, 1990; Runyan, DeVellis, DeVellis, and Hochbaum, 1982; Stone, 1987; Taylor, 1990). Since it is as yet without formal definition or consensus on name, it could be defined simply as psychologists working on public health problems. However, a more in-depth analysis shows that two basic features are emerging. First, it involves the integration and synthesis of behavioral science principles with public health and epidemiological principles, creating a more complex picture of public health phenomena. Second, it involves the extension and application of psychological theories, treatments, and research to the health problems of populations. Public health psychologists apply their knowledge not only to individuals but also to groups, organizations, communities, and societies for the purposes of obtaining and maintaining the overall health and well-being of a nation. To date, most contributions have been made in efforts to control chronic diseases, such as cancer, hypertension, and cardiovascular disease (Elder and others, 1985; McAlister, Ramirez, Galavotti, and Gallion, 1989).

Scientists from behavioral, social, health, and community psychology and from behavioral and social epidemiology have contributed most to this new applied discipline. Interventions range from traditional health education strategies to innovative strategies that incorporate live theater and video dramatizations, social marketing, and behavior modification techniques (Hovell, Elder, Blanchard, and Sallis, 1986; Rugg, Hovell, and Franzini, 1990; Tross, 1989).

Public Health Psychology's Contributions to AIDS Prevention

Since 1982, psychologists have been contributing essential information to our understanding and efforts to control the AIDS epidemic. Significant contributions have come from clinical and research psychologists focusing on the psychosocial factors surrounding HIV infection, AIDS-related complex (ARC), and the development of full-blown AIDS (Zich and Temoshok, 1987); an understanding of HIV- or AIDS-related distress and coping mechanisms (Moulton, Sweet, Temoshok, and Mandel, 1987); the extent of individual behavior change and its predictors, (Becker and Joseph, 1988; Catania and others, 1990; Coates, Stall, Catania, and Kegeles, 1988; Corby, Rhodes, Wolitski, and Kincade, 1988; Doll and others, 1990; Martin, 1987); the issues surrounding HIV counseling, testing, and test-seeking behavior (Coates, Morin, and McKusick, 1987; Rugg, Sweet, Hovell, and Fagan, 1988); experimental interventions to facilitate change in risky sexual behaviors (Kelly and St. Lawrence, 1986; Valdiserri and others, 1989a); experimental interventions to facilitate change in risky drug-using behaviors (Des Jarlais, 1989; Des Jarlais and Friedman, 1988); cultural differences in efforts to change risky behavior (Peterson and Morin, 1988); specific AIDS prevention evaluation methodologies (Leviton and Valdiserri, 1990; Rugg, O'Reilly, and Galavotti, 1990); public reactions to AIDS (Herek and Glunt, 1988); the effects of AIDS on the immune system (Kiecolt-Glaser and Glaser, 1988); neuropsychological changes seen with HIV infection in the brain (Tross and Hirsch, 1988); and the fear and stigma associated with caring for AIDS patients (Baum and Nesselhof, 1988).

More recently, psychologists have begun to play an important role in community-level interventions and media campaigns (McAlister, Ramirez, Galavotti, and Gallion, 1989). Psychologists also are making significant contributions in legislative activities (Morin, 1988).

Key Concepts in AIDS Prevention

From a public health psychology perspective, there are five key concepts that are central to understanding and preventing AIDS. The following subsections discuss each of these concepts.

A Multilevel AIDS Prevention Framework. To prevent HIV infection, we must influence risky sexual and drug-using practices, two of the most basic of human behaviors. No single discipline or one-shot intervention is going to solve this multidimensional problem; rather, a sustained, multidimensional, interdisciplinary effort with repeat exposures to a variety of well-planned and targeted strategies is essential.

A multilevel systems approach is a useful organizing framework for AIDS prevention, since so many aspects of the individual and society are currently being challenged by the epidemic and will need to be confronted before we can hope to find solutions. Such solutions need to be developed with the understanding that there will be different intervention strategies and outcome measures for each level, since each level will have different targets for change. For example, targets for change in a comprehensive HIV prevention effort might be social and cultural norms; social policies, communities; institutions, such as schools or workplaces; groups; and individuals. Individuals may be targeted in one-to-one or small-group settings, in institutions or the community, or in the society at large through national campaigns. One may also target for change the individual's specific knowledge, attitudes, or beliefs or a specific behavior. The exact intervention strategies and outcome measures will need to vary according to the sociodemographic characteristics and cultural beliefs of the target population.

It is beyond the scope of this chapter to discuss all of these levels in detail, although a comprehensive program would include as many as possible. Choosing the level on which to focus should be based on a careful analysis of the problem. Practically, this choice is often based on the time, talent, resources, and experiences of those designing the interventions. To achieve the most effective interventions, multidisciplinary teams of behavioral scientists and public health professionals are essential.

Equally important in achieving effective interventions is the implementation of extensive and well-planned evaluation activities. To help frame evaluation efforts, the intervention team should answer the following basic questions before each intervention is designed:

1. At what level is the proposed intervention targeted? (Is it the individual, the community, society, or a specific individual behavior?)
2. What specifically is expected to change? (Knowledge, attitudes, or behaviors; organizational structure or curriculum; social norms or policies?)
3. Who is the target? (What are the target population's sociodemographic, psychosocial, behavioral, and environmental characteristics?)
4. What elements should be included in the intervention? The answer to this question should be based on a careful evaluation of the answers to the first three questions, on behavioral science theory, and on past research.

Since psychologists have contributed most to individual intervention strategies, I will focus the remainder of this chapter on four concepts that are particularly relevant to AIDS prevention efforts on the individual level. The first two come from epidemiological studies; the third and fourth come from behavioral science principles.

The Stages of AIDS. Medical and epidemiological studies on AIDS have shown that there are various levels of risk and stages of infection and disease through which an individual may pass. Diagnosed cases of AIDS are the clinical end point on the continuum of infection with HIV; however, they do not necessarily reflect current HIV infection patterns, since the median interval between infection with HIV and onset of AIDS is nearly ten years (Centers for Disease Control, 1989). Projections made in May 1988 estimate that 365,000 AIDS cases will have been diagnosed in the United States by the end of 1992. Additionally, projections indicate that a total of 172,000 AIDS patients will require medical care in 1992 at a cost expected to range from $5 billion to $13 billion. These figures underestimate the true magnitude of HIV morbidity, since many clinical manifestations of HIV infection are not reportable even under the current revised AIDS case definition (Centers for Disease Control, 1989).

Epidemiological studies of HIV seroprevalence (that is, the prevalence of HIV infection as measured by the presence of HIV antibodies in the blood) in a variety of settings are currently under way (Centers for Disease Control, 1989). Such studies will help public health officials determine where to target specific interventions to control the spread of HIV. Behavioral studies will help to determine what the interventions should be.

From an intervention perspective, awareness of the different cognitive, emotional, behavioral, and personal social needs at each stage is important. For example, low-risk individuals need to have an accurate understanding of modes of transmission so that unwarranted fear and discrimination do not develop. This knowledge also may enhance their support of social programs that would facilitate change in high-risk groups. High-risk groups need interventions targeting not only behavioral change but also ways of coping with stigmatization, the threat of AIDS, and sometimes denial of risk. Those who are infected with HIV or diagnosed with AIDS need to make behavioral changes as well, but also will need additional medical, emotional, personal, and institutional support. Thus, interventions at each level may overlap, but each will require unique components.

Behavioral and social science principles can help to specify the determinants of the needs and behaviors of individuals at each stage of the disease process, and these principles can help to identify the issues and barriers to change for the target group of an intervention. Including these principles also enables specific theory-based intervention objectives to be outlined. Once objectives are clearly defined, appropriate interventions can be specified. Interventions that lack precision in their aim and clarity in their conceptualization are bound to be limited in their effectiveness.

Early epidemiological investigations helped to identify large target groups. Further behavioral epidemiological evaluation has attempted to refine the at-risk side of the process by identifying specific at-risk subgroups, defined by their behaviors; these subgroups include injection drug users and people who have frequent unprotected anal sex.

The Relative-Risk Behavioral Continuum. Epidemiological investigations of AIDS have examined a range of potential HIV transmission behaviors and found HIV to have three main modes of transmission: sexual contact with an infected person, exposure to infected blood or blood products (mainly through needle sharing among injection drug users), and perinatal transmission from an infected woman to her fetus or infant (Centers for Disease Control, 1989).

Subsequent biological and epidemiological studies are investigating the role of several factors in determining the actual risk of exposure at a given point in time for a specified behavior. Such factors as duration, frequency, and conditions of exposure (including the presence of genital ulcers), as well as the immunological competence of the host, the length of infection, and the amount of virus present in the infected partner, are all being examined.

The Relative Risk Behavioral Continuum is derived from epidemiological studies of AIDS cases and takes into account the range in relative risk for a variety of sexual and drug-using behaviors, such as unprotected intercourse, sharing needles, or oral sex. In practice, such behaviors may move up or down the continuum based on the factors just mentioned. Since behaviors exist along a continuum of risk, changing some behaviors may yield more risk reduction than others. However, the actual risk of exposure from each type of behavior also will depend on the number of partners and the background HIV seroprevalence or "pool prevalence." All of this information should be considered in targeting behavioral interventions.

Continuum of Impact Potential for AIDS Education Strategies. An important potential contribution from health psychology is the design and evaluation of AIDS education and behavior-change strategies. An understanding of how individuals initiate and sustain health behavior changes is essential if one is going to design effective behavior-change interventions. It is important to recognize that not all interventions are going to be effective, and those that are effective may need to be offered in combination with other strategies. In addition, the effects may not be immediately apparent and thus should ideally be evaluated over time. Researchers hypothesize that some interventions may have more potential for impact than others, as is suggested in Figure 1. Here printed messages alone are seen as having limited impact potential for preventing AIDS. However, when repeated frequently and in concert with a variety of other targeted strategies, they may play an important reinforcing role.

Strategies that are more likely to engage the individual completely are placed at the top of the continuum and are seen as having more potential for impact. This is based on the simple tenets that individuals have to be personally attending to the message and actively engaged before an intervention can expect to achieve an impact and that close personal contact is most likely to yield engagement consistently (Ng, Davis, Manderscheid, and Elkers, 1979). While Figure 1 is speculative and not by any means a strict ordering of strategy efficacy, it does seem to fit with current AIDS literature. Such literature (Ostrow and others, 1988; Valdiserri and others, 1989b) suggests that an important factor influencing changes in AIDS risk behaviors is having personally known someone with AIDS or with the HIV infection. Emotional as well as cognitive involvement seems to be a key factor in making AIDS personally relevant and thereby facilitating behavioral changes.

Figure 1. A Hypothetical Continuum of Psychological Involvement and Impact Potential for AIDS Education

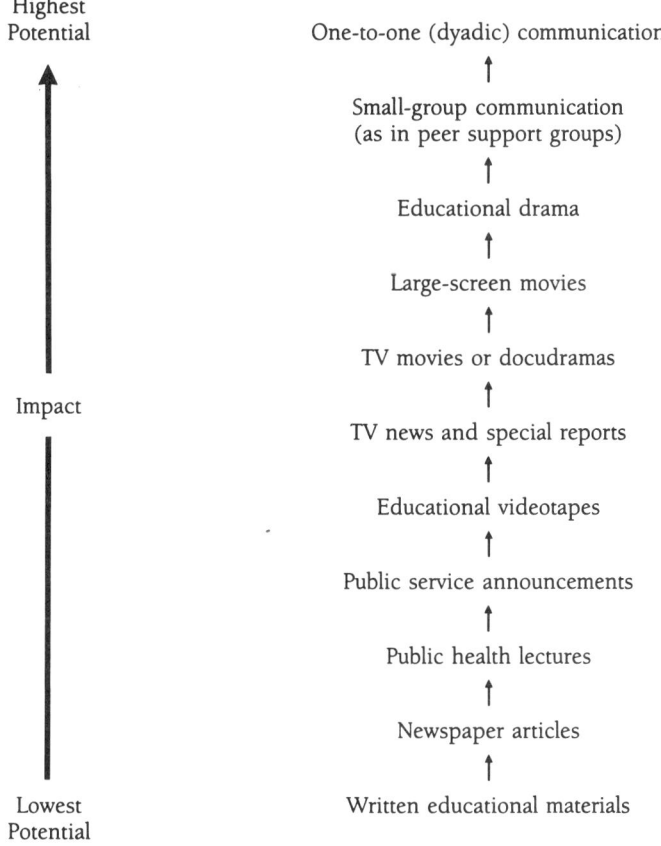

Note: Impact potential increases with repetition of the intervention.

Interventions with high potential are common in social work, counseling and clinical psychology, and in some health care transactions. However, they are relatively uncommon in health education, where information and education about disease process are emphasized as a rational basis for adopting protective behavior or discontinuing established risky behaviors (Prue, Wynder, Scharf, and Resnicow, 1987).

Strategies at the lower end of the continuum are frequently based on decision-making models that evolved out of eighteenth-century rationalism. Such models tend to see human behavior as a function of a linear reasoning process. The basic assumption is that knowledge about the potential negative consequences of one's behavior will lead to behavior change, and thus all one has to do is *inform* the individual—that is, if we provide the facts, behavior change will follow (Prue, Wynder, Scharf, and Resnicow, 1987). Unfortunately, this is often not the case.

Rather, behavioral learning theories (Bandura, 1969, 1977a, 1977b) suggest a model of health behavior and, consequently, of health behavior intervention domains where knowledge, attitude, and behavior are seen as interactional and interrelated. According to these theories, the question of causality is difficult to answer, if not unanswerable in the natural setting.

However, we can ascertain the determinants of each domain, as diagramed in Figure 2. For example, the acquisition of understandable information, one's attitudes, and the experience gained by performing a behavior are all determinants of knowledge. Persuasive communications, such as those used in social marketing strategies, plus knowledge and behaviors are determinants of attitudes (included here are most psychosocial factors such as beliefs, opinions, perceptions of norms, and efficacy). In addition to knowledge and attitudes, internal and external reinforcements are determinants of behavior.

Figure 2. Determinants of Domains for Health Promotion Interventions

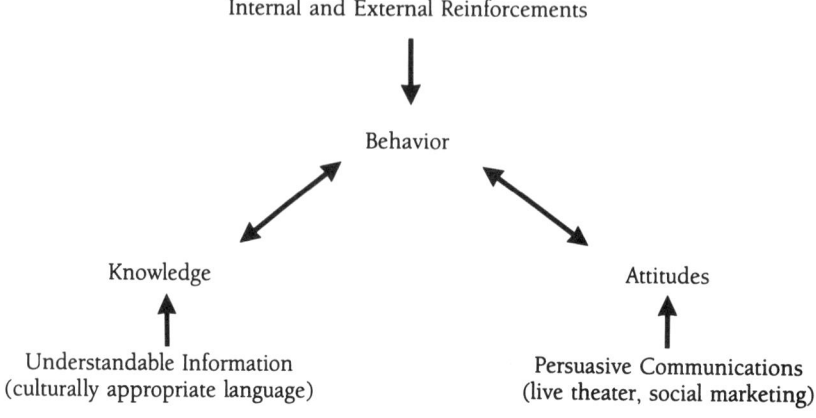

The Behavior-Change Continuum. Although the psychological literature is full of complex theories of behavior and behavior change, the Behavior-Change Continuum model suggests that most health behavior change is simply a function of behavioral change assets (that is, factors that facilitate) versus barriers (factors that hinder), where the likelihood of behavior change increases as assets increase and barriers decrease. The goal, then, is to identify and alter the barriers to change in order to enhance assets. Thus, in Figure 3, an individual's ability to make behavioral changes in seen as existing along a continuum or series of stages of "readiness to change."

Although it has a more comprehensive scope, the Behavior-Change Continuum is not at odds with any of the current AIDS risk-reduction models or frameworks offered by such investigators as Catania, Kegeles, and Coates (1990), Morin (1988), Kelly and St. Lawrence (1986), Ostrow and others (1988), and Leviton (1989). The continuum is based on the following simple tenets:

1. Individuals vary in their ability and readiness to change a behavior, and such variability exists along a continuum of readiness to change.

2. This readiness to change is a function of an individual's psychosocial, behavioral, and environmental assets versus barriers ratio, of which the individual may or may not be aware. Examples of psychosocial assets would be awareness, perceived susceptibility, efficacy, and support. Examples of behavioral assets would be having the behavioral and social skills necessary to navigate safer sex, use a condom, or clean needles and syringes. Examples of environmental assets would be the availability of condoms or clean needles or readily available drug treatment or other support services.

3. Interventions may facilitate the individual's efforts to overcome the barriers by enhancing the individual's knowledge, attitudes, beliefs, motivation, and skills and by providing support and reinforcement.

4. Interventions also may need to target environmental conditions to facilitate individual behavior change.

Although stages are suggested along this continuum, it is not a "stage theory" in the strictest sense because individuals, as hypothesized, can move back and forth along the continuum and can even skip stages. Since risky and safe behavior can exist within an individual at the same point in time, an analysis of the barriers and assets for each behavior at each point in time must be performed. For example, a female injection drug user aware of her AIDS risk and motivated to reduce her risk may find it easier to avoid sharing or to clean her "works" than to ask a male sexual partner to use a condom. She may fear punishment due to the infidelity suggested by such a request. In addition, the same woman may find it much easier to ask casual partners to use a condom, since fidelity is not an issue, but only if she is not high on drugs or alcohol. Thus, in this scenario the woman has

Figure 3. Individual Behavior-Change Model

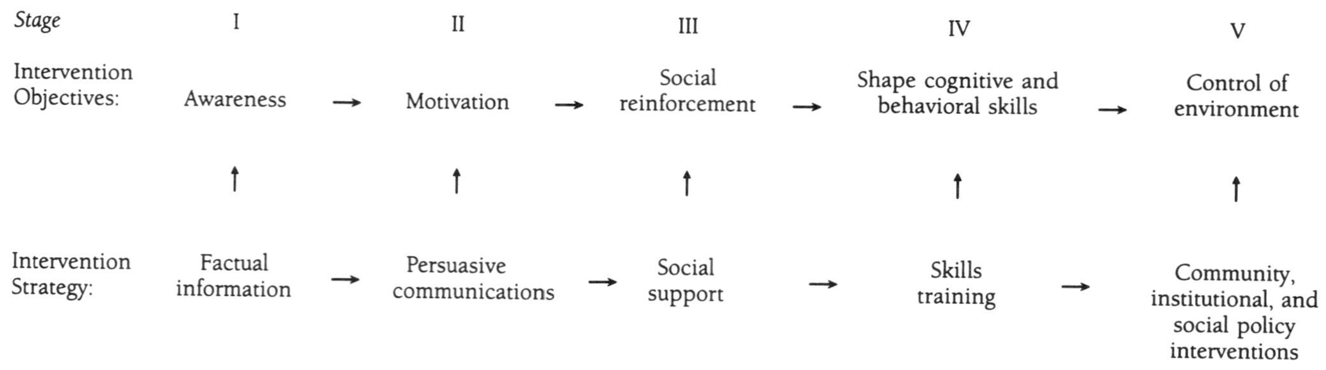

Stage	I	II	III	IV	V
Intervention Objectives:	Awareness →	Motivation →	Social reinforcement →	Shape cognitive and behavioral skills →	Control of environment
Intervention Strategy:	Factual information ↑	Persuasive communications ↑	Social support ↑	Skills training ↑	Community, institutional, and social policy interventions ↑

the awareness about AIDS and is motivated to change (awareness and motivation assets) but lacks support from her partner (a social reinforcement barrier). When she is high, she is no longer motivated and thus regresses on the continuum to the first stage. If her partner decided to try condoms one time, but they both experienced a lack of enjoyment because of the condom, then she would have awareness, motivation, and partner support, but would lack the skills to make condom use spontaneous and enjoyable (a skills barrier). Interventions for each scenario can be specified because the barrier to the performance of the behavior in each situation has been identified. Thus, this model requires a behavioral analysis for each specific situation. This analysis will allow interventions to be tailored to the individual's needs.

According to this approach, those who find it easy to change have relatively few barriers and all the psychosocial assets, behavioral skills, and environmental conditions necessary to initiate the change. For individuals in stage one, what is basically needed is an awareness about the need to change. Thus, the provision of factual information, such as the *Surgeon General's Report on AIDS* (1986) or a mass media information campaign, may be sufficient to facilitate their change.

For others, however, more may be needed. Individuals in stage two have the information and awareness about the need to change but are either denying their need to change or lack motivation. These individuals will need additional persuasive communications, such as those used in advertising and social marketing, as well as the personalized risk counseling frequently obtained in HIV counseling and testing sites, before they will be able to change.

Others will have the information and awareness, perceive that they are at risk and feel motivated to change, but still not change. For individuals in stage three, additional social supports and social reinforcements for initiating a change will be necessary. By obtaining such support, possibly through a friend, lover or peer support group, these individuals may be able to initiate a change.

Some will go through all three of these stages and still not alter their behavior. It is postulated that individuals at stage four lack the social or behavioral skills necessary to make the change. Here the actual shaping of the desired behavior will be necessary. This occurs most frequently in professionally led, multiple-session skills-training groups. However, it is possible that individuals may participate in self-help programs that teach them these skills, or that nonprofessionals will provide the training and support for skills acquisition.

Some individuals will be unable to change or to maintain change following our best intervention efforts. Many studies of gay men in longitudinal cohorts show that approximately 25 to 35 percent still participate in high-risk sexual behavior, even after exposure to multiple risk-reduction efforts (Winkelstein and others, 1987).

For individuals in stage five, environmental modifications may be the only way to facilitate their efforts to change. Examples of possible environmental alterations would be increased and enhanced drug treatment interventions, policy changes regarding needle exchange programs, the distribution of bleach bottles for needle hygiene, and the widespread distribution of condoms in the community and incentive systems for their use. The efficacy of such approaches in this country will remain speculative until sufficient evaluation research has been completed.

Clearly, enhanced environmental conditions, such as increased access to well-paying jobs, quality education, and health care, would be beneficial at each stage of the continuum. However, such global quality-of-life factors, while important, are the most difficult to affect. And since many individuals are able to make personal health behavior changes despite less than optimal social conditions, efforts should first be focused on factors more easily modified, moving up the continuum as barriers are encountered.

I offer this continuum as an organizing concept for understanding individual health risk behaviors. I have tried, as others have (Rosenstock, Strecher, and Becker, 1988), to integrate a variety of health promotion and disease prevention models and health psychological theories. This distillation of theories has yielded a model that is proving useful as a way to organize AIDS prevention activities that focus on individual behavior change. Using this model, health psychologists can place an individual, at any point in time, along this continuum for any behavior, and the appropriate intervention strategy can then be determined. Empirical tests of the model's usefulness are under way.

Recommendations for Evaluation

We will not see the end of this epidemic before coming to grips with some difficult and challenging personal and sociopolitical dilemmas. Psychologists and program evaluators from all disciplines can contribute and should be encouraged to focus immediate attention on the following agenda for evaluation research:

1. Conduct formative evaluation on screening instruments to assess individual assets and barriers.

2. Identify predictors of individual behavior change, as well as successful intervention elements, through evaluation research.

3. Evaluate what type of intervention works best for which types of individuals (in other words, evaluate "tailored interventions").

4. Evaluate innovative interventions for influencing individuals, communities, and society. Such evaluation should include strategies for determining differential effectiveness in various risk and ethnic groups.

5. Evaluate how well behavior changes are sustained over time and identify which intervention or combination of approaches is most effective in preventing relapse.

6. Conduct process evaluations to assess the extent, variability, and quality of current prevention programs and to estimate the costs, feasibility, and diffusion mechanisms for innovative strategies.

7. Work with other behavioral scientists to evaluate corroborative indicators for self-reported sexual and needle-sharing behaviors.

8. Evaluate the cost effectiveness of different interventions.

Investigators involved in this research agenda have faced many methodological constraints and difficulties. But through creativity and cross-discipline discussions of evaluation and applied research methodologies, they are formulating solutions (Turner, Miller, and Moses, 1989; Turner, Coyle, and Boruch, 1989), and study results are encouraging. For example, Kelly and St. Lawrence (1986) have shown that groups of gay men who received a multiple-session intervention based on social learning theory did significantly better in reducing risky sexual behaviors than control groups. Valdiserri and others (1989a) found that a skills-training intervention was significantly better than an education-only intervention in facilitating safer sexual behaviors in gay men. Such models need to be evaluated among bisexuals, heterosexuals, injection drug users, and minority populations as well, since most information to date has come from white gay male populations. We have learned much in a short period of time; however, many questions remain unanswered.

Conclusion

AIDS and HIV infection are not only biological events but also dramatic biopsychosocial, personal, and political phenomena. The issues they raise in disease prevention and control are complex, requiring clear thinking and the use of a multidimensional framework. The development of successful interventions requires a blending of traditional approaches from public health with innovative strategies from the behavioral sciences. Public health psychologists, program evaluators, and other behavioral scientists are uniquely poised to contribute. This multidimensional approach may be a new direction for some, and the challenges are indeed considerable, but the potential for impact is great. Only by combining public health and behavioral science principles can we expect to achieve our goals.

References

Bandura, A. *Principles of Behavior Modification*. New York: Holt, Rinehart & Winston, 1969.

Bandura, A. "Self-Efficacy: Toward a Unifying Theory of Behavior Change." *Psychological Review*, 1977a, *84*, 191-215.

Bandura, A. *Social Learning Theory.* New York: Holt, Rinehart & Winston, 1977b.
Baum, A., and Nesselhof, S.E.A. "Psychological Research and the Prevention, Etiology, and Treatment of AIDS." *American Psychologist,* 1988, *43,* 900-906.
Becker, M. H., and Joseph, J. G. "AIDS and Behavioral Change to Reduce Risk: A Review." *American Journal of Public Health,* 1988, *78* (4), 394-410.
Catania, J. A., Gibson, D. R., Marin, B., Coates, T. J., and Greenblatt, R. M. "Response Bias in Assessing Sexual Behaviors Relevant to HIV Transmission." *Evaluation and Program Planning,* 1990, *13* (1), 19-29.
Catania, J. A., Kegeles, S. M., and Coates, T. J. "Towards an Understanding of Risk Behavior: An AIDS Risk-Reduction Model (ARRM)." *Health Education Quarterly,* 1990, *17* (1), 53-72.
Centers for Disease Control. "AIDS and Human Immunodeficiency Virus Infection in the United States: 1988 Update." CDC Surveillance Supplement. *Morbidity and Mortality Weekly Report,* 1989, *38* (S-4), 1-38.
Coates, T. J., Morin, S., McKusick, L. "Behavioral Consequences of AIDS Antibody Testing Among Gay Men." *Journal of the American Medical Association,* 1987, *258,* 1889.
Coates, T. J., Stall, R. D., Catania, J. A., and Kegeles, S. M. "Behavioral Factors in the Spread of HIV Infection." *AIDS,* 1988, *2,* S239-S246.
Corby, N., Rhodes, F., Wolitski, R., and Kincade, R. L. *Predictors of HIV Serostatus at an Alternative Test Site.* Paper presented at the Fourth International Conference on AIDS, Stockholm, Sweden, June 12-16, 1988.
Des Jarlais, D. C. *Final Report for Innovative Risk-Reduction Project with Potential Intravenous Drug Users.* Atlanta, Ga.: Centers for Disease Control, 1989.
Des Jarlais, D. C., and Friedman, S. R. "The Psychology of Preventing AIDS Among Intravenous Drug Users: A Social Learning Conceptualization." *American Psychologist,* 1988, *43* (11), 865-870.
Doll, L. S., O'Malley, P., Pershing, A., Darrow, W. W., Hessol, N., and Lifson, A. "High-Risk Sexual Behavior and Knowledge of HIV Antibody Status in the San Francisco City Clinic Cohort." *Health Psychology,* 1990, *9* (3), 253-265.
Elder, J. R., Hovell, M. F., Lasater, T. M., Wells, B. L., and Carleton, R. A. "Applications of Behavior Modification to Community Health Education: The Case of Heart Disease Prevention." *Health Education Quarterly,* 1985, *12,* 151-168.
Herek, G. M., and Glunt, E. K. "An Epidemic of Stigma: Public Reactions to AIDS." *American Psychologist,* 1988, *43,* 886-891.
Hovell, M. F., Elder, J. R., Blanchard, J., and Sallis, J. F. "Behavior Analysis and Public Health Perspectives: Combining Paradigms to Effect Prevention." *Education and Treatment of Children,* 1986, *9,* 287-306.
Kelly, J. A., and St. Lawrence, J. S. "Behavioral Intervention and AIDS." *Behavior Therapist,* 1986, *6,* 121-125.
Kiecolt-Glaser, J. K., and Glaser, K. "Psychological Influences on Immunity: Implications for AIDS." *American Psychologist,* 1988, *43,* 892-898.
Leviton, L. C. "Theoretical Foundations of AIDS Prevention." In R. O. Valdiserri (ed.), *Preventing AIDS.* New Brunswick, N.J.: Rutgers University Press, 1989.
Leviton, L. C., and Valdiserri, R. O. "Evaluating AIDS Prevention: Outcome, Implementation, and Mediating Variables." *Evaluation and Program Planning,* 1990, *13* (1), 55-66.
McAlister, A., Ramirez, A. G., Galavotti, C., and Gallion, K. J. "Antismoking Campaigns: Progress in the Application of Social Learning Theory." In R. E. Rice and C. Atkin (eds.), *Public Communication Campaigns.* 2nd ed. Newbury Park, Calif.: Sage, 1989.
Martin, J. L. "The Impact of AIDS on Gay Male Sexual Behavior Patterns in New York City." *American Journal of Public Health,* 1987, *77* (5), 578-582.

Morin, S. F. "AIDS: The Challenge to Psychology." *American Psychologist,* 1988, *43* (11), 838-842.

Moulton, J. M., Sweet, D. M., Temoshok, L., and Mandel, J. S. "Attributions of Blame and Responsibility in Relation to Distress and Health Behavior Change in People with AIDS and AIDS-Related Complex." *Journal of Applied Social Psychology,* 1987, *17* (5), 493-506.

Ng, L.K.Y., Davis, D. L., Manderscheid, R. W., and Elkers, J. "Toward a Conceptual Formulation of Health and Well-Being." In P. I. Ahmed and G. V. Coelho (eds.), *Toward a New Definition of Health: Psychosocial Dimensions.* New York: Plenum, 1979.

Ostrow, D. G., Joseph, J., Soucey, J., Eller, M., Kessler, R., Phair, J., and Chmiel, J. *Mental Health and Behavioral Correlates of HIV Antibody Testing in a Cohort of Gay Men.* Paper presented at the Fourth International Conference on AIDS, Stockholm, Sweden, June 12-16, 1988.

Peterson, J. L., and Morin, G. "Issues in the Prevention of AIDS Among Black and Hispanic Men." *American Psychologist,* 1988, *43* (11), 871-877.

Prue, D. M., Wynder, E. L., Scharf, L. S., and Resnicow, K. A. "Health Education and Behavioral Analysis." *Education and Treatment of Children,* 1987, *10,* 19-32.

Rosenstock, I. M., Strecher, V. J., and Becker, M. H. "Social Learning and the Health Belief Model." *Health Education Quarterly,* 1988, *15* (2), 175-183.

Rugg, D. L., Hovell, M. F., and Franzini, L. "Behavioral Science and Public Health Perspectives: Combining Paradigms to Prevent and Control AIDS." In L. Temoshok and A. Baum (eds.), *Psychosocial Perspectives on AIDS: Etiology, Prevention, and Treatment.* Hillsdale, N.J.: Erlbaum, 1990.

Rugg, D., O'Reilly, K. R., and Galavotti, C. "AIDS Prevention Evaluation: Conceptual and Methodological Issues." *Evaluation and Program Planning,* 1990, *13* (1), 79-89.

Rugg, D., Sweet, D., Hovell, M., and Fagan, R. *Factors Affecting the Decision to Learn HIV Test Results.* Paper presented at the Fourth International Conference on AIDS, Stockholm, Sweden, June 12-16, 1988.

Runyan, C. W., DeVellis, R. F., DeVellis, B. M., and Hochbaum, G. M. "Health Psychology and the Public Health Perspective: In Search of the Pump Handle." *Health Psychology,* 1982, *1,* 169-180.

Stone, G. C. "Health Psychology in the Community Setting." In G. C. Stone (ed.), *Health Psychology: A Discipline and a Profession.* Chicago: University of Chicago Press, 1987.

Stone, G. C., Cohen, F., Adler, N. E., and Associates. *Health Psychology—A Handbook: Theories, Applications, and Challenges of a Psychological Approach to the Health Care System.* San Francisco: Jossey-Bass, 1979.

Surgeon General's Report on Acquired Immune Deficiency Syndrome. Washington, D.C.: U.S. Department of Health and Human Services, 1986.

Taylor, S. E. "Health Psychology: The Science and the Field." *American Psychologist,* 1990, *45,* 40-50.

Tross, S. *Psychological Skills Training/Media Program to Decrease AIDS Risk Behavior: Final Report.* Atlanta, Ga.: Centers for Disease Control, 1989.

Tross, S., and Hirsch, D. A. "Psychological Distress and Neurological Complications of HIV Infection and AIDS." *American Psychologist,* 1988, *43,* 929-934.

Turner, C. F., Coyle, S., and Boruch, R. *Evaluating AIDS Prevention Programs.* Washington, D.C.: National Research Council, National Academy Press, 1989.

Turner, C. F., Miller, H. G., and Moses, L. E. (eds.). *AIDS: Sexual Behavior and Intravenous Drug Use.* Washington, D.C.: National Research Council, 1989.

Valdiserri, R. O., Lyter, D. W., Leviton, L. C., Callahan, C. M., Kingsley, L. A., and Rinaldo, C. R. "AIDS Prevention in Homosexual and Bisexual Men: Results of a Randomized Trial Evaluating Two Risk-Reduction Interventions." *AIDS,* 1989a, *3,* 21-26.

Valdiserri, R. O., Lyter, D. W., Leviton, L. C., Callahan, C. M., Kingsley, L. A., and Rinaldo, C. R. "Variables Influencing Condom Use in a Cohort of Gay and Bisexual Men." *American Journal of Public Health*, 1989b, 78, 801-805.

Winkelstein, W., Lyman, D. M., Padian, N., Grant, R., Samuel, M., Wiley, J. A., Anderson, R. E., Lang, W., Riggs, J., and Levy, J. A. "Sexual Practices and Risk of Infection by the Human Immunodeficiency Virus." *Journal of the American Medical Association*, 1987, 257, 321-325.

Zich, J., and Temoshok, L. "Perceptions of Social Support in Men with AIDS and ARC: Relationships with Distress and Hardiness." *Journal of Applied Social Psychology*, 1987, 17 (3), 193-215.

Deborah L. Rugg is a research psychologist in the Behavioral and Prevention Research Branch, Division of Sexually Transmitted Diseases, Centers for Disease Control.

A variety of motivations exist for constructing mathematical models of the AIDS epidemic, including forecasting, scientific estimation of disease parameters, and policy analysis. This chapter discusses several different modeling approaches and their attendant uses, stressing the results most relevant to policy analysts and program evaluators.

An Overview of AIDS Modeling

Edward H. Kaplan

A growing number of researchers are constructing mathematical models of the AIDS epidemic. As the cumulative U.S. AIDS caseload approaches 150,000 and because over 80,000 people have died of AIDS in the United States (Centers for Disease Control, 1990), it is natural to ask how many more AIDS cases and deaths will ensue over the years ahead, both in the United States and abroad. Mathematical models can provide a reasonable approach to producing such forecasts.

Models can also help us understand the properties and natural progression of AIDS. For example, proliferation of the AIDS virus depends on biological quantities, such as AIDS incubation times and conditional transmission probabilities, that cannot be observed directly. Models allow researchers to estimate these quantities indirectly from available data.

Perhaps most important, AIDS models suggest necessary conditions for ending the AIDS epidemic and highlight the amount of time required for significant changes to occur. Incorporating the key features of proposed intervention programs into such models can provide analysts with a powerful approach to program evaluation. Doing so can only sharpen the debate about such controversial policies as condom distribution in schools, widespread HIV testing, and needle exchange.

This chapter provides an overview of AIDS modeling to date, emphasizing those techniques and results that provide the greatest insight to policy analysts and program evaluators.

Forecasting Models

The need for AIDS forecasts is obvious; planners require estimates of future caseloads for determining health care requirements and costs. Statistical forecasting models produce short-run predictions of AIDS caseloads based on past trends. Here we will consider three different approaches that have been employed.

Statisticians at the U.S. Centers for Disease Control (CDC) have employed maximum-likelihood estimation to estimate the future numbers of AIDS cases in the United States, both in the aggregate and by various subgroups, such as those determined by geographic subdivision or risk status. Define A_t as the number of AIDS cases reported during time t after adjusting for reporting delays (see Downs and others, 1988; Heisterkamp and others, 1988; or Karon, Devine, and Morgan, 1989 for proposed adjustment methods). The CDC formulation employs the Box-Cox transformation, which yields the following model:

$$\frac{A_t^\omega - 1}{\omega} = \beta_0 + \beta_1 t + \beta_2 t^2 + \beta_3 t^3 \ldots + \beta_k t^k + \epsilon_t \qquad (1)$$

where ω and β_0 through β_k are parameters to be estimated and the ϵ_t is an error term. The Box-Cox parameter ω serves to transform the observed caseloads to match the observed time trends best; for example, as ω approaches zero, the left-hand side of equation 1 approaches $\log(A_t)$. In producing published forecasts, k has typically been set to one or two (Karon, Devine, and Morgan, 1989). As reported widely, the CDC has projected a cumulative U.S. AIDS caseload of 365,000 by the end of 1992 using this method (Heyward and Curran, 1988), while more recent work by Karon, Devine, and Morgan (1989) suggests that this figure could be higher.

A simpler approach has been reported by researchers from the Los Alamos National Laboratory. Letting C_t represent the cumulative count of AIDS cases reported to the CDC (unadjusted for reporting delays), Hyman and Stanley (1988) showed that

$$\hat{C}_t = 174.6(t - 1981.2)^3 + 340 \qquad (2)$$

provides a good approximation to C_t (within $\pm 2\%$). Plotting the cube root of observed cumulative AIDS caseloads versus time yields straight lines when the data are examined by geographic region and by risk groups. Thus, a "quick-and-dirty" approach to short-run forecasting in a given situation is to collect the relevant C_t data (preferably adjusting the reporting delays) and to fit the model

$$C_t^{1/3} = \beta_0 + \beta_1 t + \epsilon_t \qquad (3)$$

via regression. This approach is analogous to the Box-Cox method with $\omega = 1/2$ and $k = 1$ (for if the cube root of C_t is linear over time, then the square root of A_t should be roughly linear as well).

A third approach, called "back calculation," has been suggested by Brookmeyer and Gail (1988). This approach relies on the availability of an estimated probability distribution for the AIDS incubation time—that is, the time from initial HIV infection to manifestation of AIDS. Such incubation time distributions are available from studies of blood transfusion recipients (Medley, Anderson, Cox, and Billard, 1987) and cohorts of gay men (Lui, Darrow, and Rutherford, 1988; Bacchetti and Moss, 1989). Let $I(x)$ equal the rate at which new HIV infections occur at time x and $f(x)$ be the incubation time probability density function. By definition, then, the rate at which AIDS cases occur at time t, $A(t)$, is given by the convolution

$$A(t) = \int_0^t I(x) f(t - x) \, dx. \tag{4}$$

Now, by assumption, the probability density $f(x)$ is known, while the AIDS case rate $A(t)$ can be set equal to A_t (again, following adjustment for reporting delays). As shown by Brookmeyer and Gail (1988), the function $I(x)$ can be approximated from equation 4 using available data. Once $I(x)$ has been estimated, the cumulative AIDS caseload by some future time τ is found from

$$C(\tau) = \int_0^\tau \hat{A}(t) \, dt \tag{5}$$

where $\hat{A}(t)$ is found from equation 4 using the estimated infection rate function $\hat{I}(x)$.

Brookmeyer and Gail (1988) have employed this model to place a lower bound on the magnitude of the AIDS epidemic in the United States by assuming that $I(x)$ dropped to zero as of the start of 1987 and allowing τ to approach infinity in equation 5. For example, using a Weibull distribution with a mean of eight years to describe the incubation time produced a lower bound of 366,000 cumulative AIDS cases.

Of the three approaches discussed, the "cube-root law" advanced by Hyman and Stanley (1988) certainly provides the simplest method, while the back-calculation model requires the most computational effort. For short forecasting intervals, the methods are not likely to differ greatly in their projections (Heyward and Curran, 1988). Over longer time frames, however, it seems clear that the back-calculation approach has the potential to provide better forecasts due to its incorporation of the natural progression of AIDS. In particular, back calculation can include better information regarding the AIDS incubation time distribution as such information becomes available; extrapolation methods do not stand to gain from similar advances in data collection. Other statistical models not discussed here may be found in the work of Pickering and others (1988), Richardson, Caroni, and Papaevangelou (1988), and Taylor (1989).

Modeling HIV Transmission Dynamics

Statistical models based on extrapolating past trends, though potentially accurate, do not offer explanations of why the AIDS epidemic has progressed (or is progressing) as observed or of how the epidemic might change in response to behavior modifications or policy interventions. To understand these issues requires a more sophisticated approach that relates the key features of the epidemic (HIV transmission via risky behavior, the progression of disease from HIV infection through AIDS, and natural population dynamics) to the number of HIV infections and AIDS cases that occur over time. As we will show, even the simplest HIV transmission models contain lessons of great import to policy analysts and program evaluators; such models, in effect, demonstrate what must occur to end the AIDS epidemic. What follows is a deliberately oversimplified derivation to illustrate the key insight that emerges from HIV transmission models; more realistic results will be summarized afterward.

Consider the following model of a population of gay men at risk for HIV infection (and hence AIDS); this model is a simplification of the arguments found in Anderson, Medley, May, and Johnson (1986), May and Anderson (1987), and Kaplan (1989c). An average of N men per year join this population (thus, N is the arrival or recruitment rate). In the absence of HIV or AIDS, men remain in this population for an average of $1/\mu$ years; we assume for simplicity that this residence time in an uninfected population is exponentially distributed. Men in the population are assumed to engage in various risky sexual activities, such as unprotected anal sex. Let λ denote the mean number of risky sex partners per year for a randomly chosen man in this population (thus, λ is the risky sex rate). When an uninfected man is exposed to HIV via risky sex with an infected man, the uninfected man is assumed to become infected with probability ι (for infectivity). Manifestation of AIDS occurs on average $1/\gamma$ years past infection with HIV ($1/\gamma$ is the mean incubation time); again, for simplicity we assume an exponential distribution over the AIDS incubation times. Denoting the number of uninfected and infected men in the population at time t by $U(t)$ and $I(t)$, respectively, these assumptions imply the following pair of differential equations:

$$\frac{dU(t)}{dt} = N - \left[\lambda \iota \frac{I(t)}{U(t) + I(t)} + \mu\right] U(t), \qquad (6)$$

$$\frac{dI(t)}{dt} = \left[\lambda \iota \frac{U(t)}{U(t) + I(t)} - (\mu + \gamma)\right] I(t). \qquad (7)$$

In conjunction with initial conditions, equations 6 and 7 specify the course of an HIV/AIDS epidemic under the assumptions stated; the rate at which AIDS cases occur at time t simply equals $\gamma I(t)$.

Consider the situation early in the epidemic when virtually all men are uninfected. During this time period, the ratio $U(t)/[U(t) + I(t)]$ essentially equals one; thus equation 7 simplifies to the following exponential growth (or decay) model:

$$\frac{dI(t)}{dt} \cong \left[\lambda \iota - (\mu + \gamma) \right] I(t) \quad \text{(when } I(t) \text{ is small)} \tag{8}$$

Clearly, the number of infected men will increase if and only if the term $\lambda \iota - (\mu + \gamma)$ is positive. Restating this relation, we see that an epidemic will develop if and only if

$$R_0 = \frac{\lambda \iota}{\mu + \gamma} > 1. \tag{9}$$

The term R_0 is known as the reproductive rate of infection (Anderson, Medley, May, and Johnson, 1986; May and Anderson, 1987; Kaplan, 1989c) and represents the number of infections generated directly by a newly infected man early in the epidemic. The threshold condition of equation 9 states that in order for an epidemic to occur, the number of infections generated by a newly infected man must exceed one, for the infected man must replace himself by more than one infected person on average for the infection to propagate in the population.

The fundamental task in attempting to control HIV and AIDS, then, is to reduce the magnitude of R_0 below unity. Equation 9 is remarkable in this light, for it states that λ, the risky sex rate, need not approach zero for AIDS to be eliminated; as we will argue later, this implies that behavioral modification programs such as safe-sex education need not be perfect to be effective. Alternatively, the infectivity ι need not approach zero; this implies that interventions that impact on infectivity (such as condom use or a vaccine) need not be perfect as well. We will return to such arguments in the next section of this chapter, but now we must address the fact that the model considered thus far oversimplifies reality. The existence and import of a threshold result similar to equation 9, however, remain even under complex model formulations.

There are several aspects of the model discussed that can be made more realistic. For example, note the assumption that all men average λ risky sex partners per year. Of course, there will be those who average many sex partners, those with few, and those with intermediate numbers. To accommodate this, we may consider variable risky sex rates. Thus, the numbers of uninfected and infected men with risky sex rate λ can be denoted by $U(\lambda)$ and $I(\lambda)$, respectively, but λ is now free to vary over some range. Similarly, the arrival rate can be indexed by the risky sex rate of the newly arriving man, yielding several arrival rates of the form $N(\lambda)$. However, once we have stratified the population by risky sex rates, it becomes necessary to specify how men with different sex drives mix.

At one extreme, it might be assumed that no mixing occurs across different sexual activity levels. In such a segregated environment, equation 9 applies separately to each of the different risky sex strata; epidemics would only develop for those with $\lambda > (\mu + \gamma)/\iota$. Another extreme is to assume random (or proportionate) mixing across subgroups. In this instance, a threshold similar to equation 9 holds. As argued by Anderson, Medley, May, and Johnson (1986) and May and Anderson (1987), the effective value for λ to use in equation 9, λ_{eff} is

$$\lambda_{\text{eff}} = \text{Mean}(\lambda) + \frac{\text{Variance}(\lambda)}{\text{Mean}(\lambda)}. \tag{10}$$

Equation 10 reflects the disproportionate role played by those with the highest risky sex rates in the population. As λ_{eff} exceeds the mean risky sex rate, random-mixing epidemics can occur even when the mean risky sex rate is less than $(\mu + \gamma)/\iota$.

Of course, segregation and random mixing are but two of many mixing possibilities across risky sex rates. More sophisticated models that allow for various nonrandom mixing patterns can be found in the work of Abramson and Rothschild (1988), Hyman and Stanley (1988), Jacquez and others (1988), Kaplan, Cramton, and Paltiel (1989), Koopman and others (1988), and May and Anderson (1988). All of these models, though perhaps more complicated mathematically than equation 9, possess threshold results that bear the same implications for policy analysts.

In presenting equations 6 and 7, we assumed that both the residence time in the population (without regard to HIV or AIDS) and the AIDS incubation time followed exponential distributions. Neither of these assumptions is necessary; it is possible to construct models with more realistic distributions. For example, the distribution of the AIDS incubation time has been estimated as approximately Weibull or gamma in shape (Lui, Darrow, and Rutherford, 1988; Medley, Anderson, Cox, and Billard, 1987). Kaplan (1989c) presents a formula for the reproductive rate of infection assuming arbitrary probability distributions for the residence and AIDS incubation times under the assumption of random mixing, while the threshold formulation in Kaplan, Cramton, and Paltiel (1989) allows arbitrary probability distributions and arbitrary nonrandom mixing across different risky sex strata in the population. In addition, the latter threshold allows infectivity to depend on sexual practice (for example, the differential risks of receptive versus insertive anal intercourse).

A note on infectivity is in order. Most HIV transmission models assume that infectivity is best applied per partner as opposed to per sex act. Recent research indicates that per-partner infectivity better approximates the relations found empirically between the number of sex acts, number of sex partners, and incident infections (Grant, Wiley, and Winkelstein, 1987; May, Anderson, and Blower, 1989; Kaplan, 1990; Wiley, Herschkorn, and Padian, 1989). Also, recent evidence suggests that infectivity varies over the course of the AIDS incubation period (Anderson and May, 1988; Hyman and Stanley, 1988). Though this certainly complicates HIV transmission models, the fundamental threshold result still remains (with an appropriately averaged infectivity appearing in the formula for the reproductive rate).

Finally, the model presented earlier and the generalizations discussed to this point apply only to gay men, yet there are others at risk for AIDS, notably intravenous drug users who share injection equipment and sexually active heterosexuals. Kaplan (1989b) has constructed a simple model of HIV transmission via shared injection equipment and has shown how policies such as needle or bleach distribution can affect the epidemic. A threshold condition for heterosexual epidemics was presented by May and Anderson (1987), while Dietz (1988) has extended this model to account for the duration of heterosexual relationships. As argued earlier, one can construct, in principle, HIV transmission models of arbitrary complexity, but the existence of a threshold condition that determines when epidemics can and cannot occur remains the most important result. Let us now turn to the policy implications of HIV transmission models.

Policy Models

Policy analysts are often faced with the task of evaluating proposed intervention measures, while program evaluators are called on to determine the performance of implemented programs. Both of these tasks can benefit from the insights provided by HIV transmission models. Policy models can suggest necessary conditions for a proposed intervention to succeed and estimate the time frame necessary for the effects of the intervention to become apparent. These models also suggest important performance measures for program evaluation and can help forecast long-run program performance consistent with current observations.

The basic idea in policy modeling is to incorporate the features of an intervention program in an HIV transmission model. How this is done is largely dependent on the nature of the program being evaluated and on the specifics of HIV transmission dynamics in the situation under consideration (for example, sexual transmission, IV transmission via shared injection equipment, transfusion, or any combination of these). Several examples will now be presented.

Safer Sex. A goal of any program addressing sexually transmitted HIV is to reduce the risky sex rates of those in the population under study. Using data from San Francisco, Kaplan (1989c) examined the reductions in HIV prevalence and the AIDS case rate over time that would occur due to reductions in risky sex rates among gay men corresponding to the following assumptions: The AIDS incubation time follows a Weibull distribution with a mean of eight years (Lui, Darrow, and Rutherford, 1988; Medley, Anderson, Cox, and Billard, 1987); gay men remain sexually active in the absence of the HIV or AIDS for an average of thirty-two years (May and Anderson, 1987); infectivity averages 0.075 per partner (as derived using the data of Grant, Wiley, and Winkelstein, 1987); currently, 50 percent of the population is infected with HIV (Grant, Wiley, and Winkelstein, 1987); risky sex rates are distributed geometrically; and partners are selected at random. Kaplan showed that even under conditions of abstinence from risky sex, it would take over twenty years for the AIDS case rate to dwindle to negligible levels. Using a result analogous to equation 9, he also showed that a reduction to an average of 1.46 risky sex partners per year or fewer would eventually eliminate AIDS, although after twenty-five years, 10 percent of the population studied would still remain infected with HIV.

In a different study, Kaplan and Abramson (1989) explicitly accounted for a reported problem with sex education programs: Some men who modify their behavior due to an educational intervention in time relapse into risky sexual practices. Kaplan and Abramson assume that in the absence of the intervention, the epidemic progresses in a manner similar, but not identical, to equations 6 and 7. However, on implementation of the program, sexually active men are assumed to withdraw from risky sex at per-capita rate ϵ (per year), while men who are abstaining from risky sex relapse at per-capita rate ρ (per year). Kaplan and Abramson show that the reproductive rate of infection depends on the recidivism and withdrawal rates and that even if recidivistic behavior is certain (as implied by this model), it is possible to reduce the reproductive rate below unity by increasing the withdrawal rate, reducing the recidivism rate, modifying the average risky sex rate, or any combination of these actions. Thus, though such a program is not perfect—there are always men practicing risky sex—it can conceivably eliminate HIV infection.

Screening for HIV Infection. One AIDS containment policy that has been hotly debated is HIV screening. Gail, Preston, and Piantadosi (1989) have developed a model that incorporates the workings of a voluntary confidential screening program into the transmission dynamics of HIV. Essentially, these researchers assume that an infected person who receives a positive test result will modify his or her behavior in such a way that on average, the person will present a lower risk of infection to an uninfected partner (for example, via insistence on protected sex). The model incorporates the possibilities of both false-positive and false-negative test results. One key performance measure considered is the economic ratio, which is defined as the number of HIV tests required to prevent one AIDS case. Gail, Preston, and Piantadosi show that voluntary confidential testing can prevent large numbers of infections in isolated high-prevalence groups, yielding low values of the economic ratio. Alternatively, such testing in isolated low-prevalence populations yields some benefits but at high cost (as measured by the economic ratio). In a simulation of a mixed population, the researchers found that targeting screening toward the higher-risk groups performed better than equal screening effort across all risk groups.

Containing IV-Spread HIV Transmission. Kaplan (1989b) has developed a model that traces the development of an HIV/AIDS epidemic where the infection is spread via shared drug injection equipment. This analysis differs from the models discussed thus far, for the epidemic is viewed from the perspective of a needle rather than the perspective of a person. It is argued that sharing injection equipment leads to more rapid epidemic spread than does sexual transmission; this assertion is shown to be consistent with data from the northeast United States. Kaplan's model leads to an expression for the reproductive rate of infection that depends on the per-addict mean and mean-squared injection equipment sharing rate; the ratio of addicts to injection kits (needles and "works") in the population; the infectivity of HIV via shared injection equipment; the likelihood that infectious equipment is "flushed" clean on use by an uninfected addict; and the inactivation rate of HIV (such as the rate at which HIV perishes within a syringe). The model is also modified to consider the effect of imperfect bleaching of injection equipment.

Through examination of the formula for the reproductive rate, Kaplan shows that needle distribution (corresponding to decreasing the addict-to-needle ratio), bleach distribution, reduction in sharing rates, or any combination of these could retard or eliminate an IV-spread HIV epidemic. Needle exchange may also be considered within this framework, since exchanging an infectious needle for a clean needle is equivalent to inactivation of HIV within the needle being exchanged. For a given mean injection equipment sharing rate, these control measures have greater impact in populations with low variability in sharing rates. Also, though it seems possible to control HIV transmission in the manners suggested, it is still true that "nothing happens overnight"; reducing the prevalence of HIV may require several years.

An Imperfect Immunizing Vaccine. No vaccine has been developed for HIV infection, nor does it appear that one will be developed quickly. Still, it is reasonable to query how effective a vaccine must be in order to eliminate AIDS if such a vaccine were to be produced and administered. Kaplan (1989c) shows that the reproductive rate of infection in the presence of an immunizing vaccine equals the product of the original reproductive rate and the vaccine failure probability. Thus, the vaccine failure rate cannot exceed the reciprocal of the original reproductive rate if AIDS is to be eliminated in time. Again focusing on data from San Francisco, Kaplan argues that a vaccine must be at least 79 percent effective to eliminate AIDS. Kaplan also shows that AIDS would diminish much more quickly in the presence of an imperfect vaccine than it would due to an equivalent reduction in risky sex rates. He argues that this is due to two benefits: direct protection of those successfully vaccinated and indirect protection of those not successfully vaccinated, for the sex partners of this latter group would contain some who have been successfully vaccinated, thus reducing the likelihood that such a partner is infected.

There are two recurring themes in the previous examples. The first, as emphasized throughout this chapter, is that programs need not be perfect to end the AIDS epidemic. A perfect program is defined as an intervention that halts all transmission of HIV. One cannot readily expect proposed or implemented programs to survive this definition of perfect, although the implementation of laboratory screening of donated blood comes the closest. Therefore, it is somewhat reassuring to note that some degree of program imperfection can occur and the program can still act to eliminate HIV and AIDS over time.

The second theme, of course, is that changes in the epidemic will take time, even under unduly optimistic conditions, such as abstinence from risky activity or the development of a perfect vaccine. Evaluators should note, then, that changes in HIV prevalence and the AIDS case rate will not occur rapidly, even for highly effective programs. Changes in the number of new HIV infections, however, are more likely to be noticed over the short run. Thus, empirical studies would do well to focus on the rate of new infections as opposed to the number (or percentage) of infected persons (or AIDS cases) in a population.

Adverse Behavioral Response

Perhaps the most glaring omission from the models discussed here is the fact that these models do not account for adverse behavioral change in response to implemented interventions. The pursuit of risky activities may increase if the perceived risk of these activities decreases. Thus, though the danger of any individual risky act may decrease, the overall reduction in HIV transmission will be less than expected due to adverse behavioral response. For example, individuals who do not currently pursue IV drug usage might experiment in response to a needle distribution program— hence the fear that such programs could lead to increases in the number of drug addicts in society (Kleiman and Mockler, 1988).

Some might argue that a correct answer to this question requires an experiment in which one might assess the behavioral response of addicts to clean needles or teenagers to condom accessibility, for example. Others might argue that behavioral response concerns are politically motivated, and I would agree that many who argue for or against control policies, such as needle exchange and sex education, do so for political as opposed to scientific reasons. The approach suggested here is as follows: First, determine the benefits from a proposed intervention (using a policy model) assuming no adverse behavioral response. Then, determine the degree of adverse behavioral change necessary to destroy all of these benefits, and ask whether such changes are likely to occur. In the absence of data describing actual behavioral change, this approach can be persuasive, especially if the requisite amount of behavioral change necessary to eradicate program benefits is very large or very small.

Consider the following deliberately simplified example. Ignoring heterogeneity in risky sex rates, imagine that a particular group (such as teenagers) averages λ risky sex partners per unit time. If the likelihood that a selected sex partner is infected is denoted by π (for prevalence) and if ι represents the infectivity due to HIV exposure via risky sex, then current sexual practice in the population implies an infection rate of $\lambda \iota \pi$ per susceptible person per unit time in this population. Now suppose that condoms are distributed in conjunction with a safe-sex program. Given the reliability of condoms and the fraction of time they are used correctly, suppose that the infectivity ι is reduced to some quantity $\iota^* = \alpha \iota$, where in some sense α represents the condom failure or misuse probability over the course of a sexual relationship and, for simplicity, is assumed independent of λ. To keep the infection rate equivalent in the population would require adverse behavioral response that increases λ to $\lambda^* = \lambda/\alpha$ (for then $\lambda^* \iota^* \pi = \lambda/\alpha \cdot \alpha \iota \cdot \pi = \lambda \iota \pi$ as before). So, if α equals 10 percent, then the risky sex rate would have to increase by at least a factor of ten for the program to prove ineffective. It is hard to imagine such a drastic increase in the risky sex rate.

The logic of this example can be extended to more realistic situations. Suppose that one could demonstrate that the benefits of needle distribution or exchange would survive if the size of the addict population increased by a factor less than two. As it is difficult to imagine a doubling of the addict population, this result should instill confidence in a policy maker considering the implementation of such a scheme. Alternatively, if the benefits of the program are easily slighted by a small increase in the addict population, then it becomes difficult to argue for the program. As the public debate surrounding controversial AIDS intervention programs continues, calculations such as those suggested here can serve to inform parties on both sides of the issues.

Conclusion

Mathematical models can contribute to a better understanding of the AIDS epidemic's past, present, and future. Status-quo projections can be obtained from simple forecasting models, as described earlier in this chapter, while the likely impact of alternative policy interventions can be ascertained from policy models of HIV transmission. Regarding policy models, note that all of the examples presented here rely on relatively simple formulations of HIV transmission dynamics. To the extent that descriptive accuracy is desired, one might argue that more complicated models incorporating nonrandom mixing, variable infectivity, and behavioral modification should be applied. However, data for more complicated formulations are lacking. For example, it is difficult enough to assess the sexual activity of a given person, let alone the sexual activity for each of the partners of that same person (Abramson, 1988). Furthermore, policy analysts in any given circumstance should be concerned with the worst case. Surely the relative cost of underestimating the number of infected persons outweighs the relative cost of overestimation! In this light, it is reassuring to note that simple models of HIV transmission appear to provide an upper bound on the number of infections. For example, Kaplan, Cramton, and Paltiel (1989) examined a number of alternative mixing formulations and discovered that in circumstances leading to epidemic spread, random mixing tended to provide an upper bound for the total number infected. More recently, Kaplan (1989a) has considered a circumstance where an analyst who erroneously assumes random mixing in a segregated sexual environment still reaches an appropriate policy conclusion; this is demonstrated by examining the worst epidemic possible under segregation.

The important lesson, then, is that appropriate policy decisions appear to be much more robust to the specifics of HIV transmission models than the actual predicted numbers of uninfected and infected persons arising from these models would suggest. The complexity of a model employed for policy analysis should be limited by data that are available and obtainable and by the decisions for which the model will be used (Brandt, 1989).

References

Abramson, P. R. "Sexual Assessment and the Epidemiology of AIDS." *Journal of Sex Research*, 1988, 25 (3), 323-346.

Abramson, P. R., and Rothschild, B. "Sex, Drugs, and Matrices: Mathematical Prediction of HIV Infection." *Journal of Sex Research*, 1988, 25 (1), 106-122.

Anderson, R. M., and May, R. M. "Epidemiological Parameters of HIV Transmission." *Nature*, 1988, 333, 514-519.

Anderson, R. M., Medley, G. F., May, R. M., and Johnson, A. M. "A Preliminary

Study of the Transmission Dynamics of the Human Immunodeficiency Virus (HIV), the Causative Agent of AIDS." *IMA Journal of Mathematics Applied in Medicine and Biology,* 1986, 3, 229-263.

Bacchetti, P., and Moss, A. R. "Incubation Period of AIDS in San Francisco." *Nature,* 1989, 338, 251-253.

Brandt, E. N. "Policy Implications of Modeling of the AIDS Epidemic." *Statistics in Medicine,* 1989, 8 (1), 137-139.

Brookmeyer, R., and Gail, M. H. "A Method for Obtaining Short-Term Projections and Lower Bounds on the Size of the AIDS Epidemic." *Journal of the American Statistical Association,* 1988, 83 (402), 301-308.

Centers for Disease Control. *HIV/AIDS Surveillance Report.* Atlanta, Ga.: Centers for Disease Control, June 1990.

Dietz, K. "The Dynamics of Spread of HIV in the Heterosexual Population." In J. C. Jager and E. J. Ruitenberg (eds.), *Statistical Analysis and Mathematical Modeling of AIDS.* Oxford, England: Oxford University Press, 1988.

Downs, A. M., Ancelle, R. A., Jager, J. C., Heisterkamp, S. H., van Druten, J.A.M., Ruitenberg, E. J., and Brunet, J. B. "The Statistical Estimation, from Routine Surveillance Data, of Past, Present, and Future Trends in AIDS Incidence in Europe." In J. C. Jager and E. J. Ruitenberg (eds.), *Statistical Analysis and Mathematical Modeling of AIDS.* Oxford, England: Oxford University Press, 1988.

Gail, M. H., Preston, D., and Piantadosi, S. "Disease Prevention Models of Voluntary Confidential Screening for Human Immunodeficiency Virus (HIV)." *Statistics in Medicine,* 1989, 8 (1), 59-81.

Grant, R., Wiley, J., and Winkelstein, W. "Infectivity of the Human Immunodeficiency Virus: Estimates from a Prospective Study of Homosexual Men." *Journal of Infectious Diseases,* 1987, 156 (1), 189-193.

Heisterkamp, S. H., Jager, J. C., Downs, A. M., van Druten, J.A.M., and Ruitenberg, E. J. "Statistical Estimation of AIDS Incidence from Surveillance Data and the Link with Modeling of Trends." In J. C. Jager and E. J. Ruitenberg (eds.), *Statistical Analysis and Mathematical Modeling of AIDS.* Oxford, England: Oxford University Press, 1988.

Heyward, W. L., and Curran, J. W. "The Epidemiology of AIDS in the U.S." *Scientific American,* 1988, 259 (4), 72-81.

Hyman, J. M., and Stanley, E. A. "Using Mathematical Models to Understand the AIDS Epidemic." *Mathematical Biosciences,* 1988, 90, 415-473.

Jacquez, J. A., Simon, C. P., Koopman, J., Sattenspiel, L., and Parry, T. "Modeling and Analyzing HIV Transmission: The Effect of Contact Patterns." *Mathematical Biosciences,* 1988, 92, 119-199.

Kaplan, E. H. "Can Bad Models Suggest Good Policies? Sexual Mixing and the AIDS Epidemic." *Journal of Sex Research,* 1989a, 26 (3), 301-314.

Kaplan, E. H. "Needles That Kill: Modeling Human Immunodeficiency Virus Transmission via Shared Drug Injection Equipment in Shooting Galleries." *Reviews of Infectious Diseases,* 1989b, 11 (2), 289-298.

Kaplan, E. H. "What Are the Risks of Risky Sex? Modeling the AIDS Epidemic." *Operations Research,* 1989c, 37 (2), 198-209.

Kaplan, E. H. "Modeling HIV Infectivity: Must Sex Acts Be Counted?" *Journal of Acquired Immune Deficiency Syndromes,* 1990, 3 (1), 55-61.

Kaplan, E. H., and Abramson, P. R. "So What If the Program Ain't Perfect? A Mathematical Model of AIDS Education." *Evaluation Review,* 1989, 13 (2), 107-122.

Kaplan, E. H., Cramton, P. C., and Paltiel, A. D. "Nonrandom Mixing Models of HIV Transmission." In C. Castillo-Chavez (ed.), *Mathematical and Statistical*

Approaches to AIDS Epidemiology. Lecture Notes in Biomathematics, no. 83. Berlin: Springer-Verlag, 1989.

Karon, J. M., Devine, O. J., and Morgan, W. M. "Predicting AIDS Incidence by Extrapolating from Recent Trends." In C. Castillo-Chavez (ed.), *Mathematical and Statistical Approaches to AIDS Epidemiology. Lecture Notes in Biomathematics,* no. 83. Berlin: Springer-Verlag, 1989.

Kleiman, M.A.R., and Mockler, R. A. *AIDS and Heroin: Strategies for Control.* Washington, D.C.: Urban Institute, 1988.

Koopman, J., Simon, C., Jacquez, J., Joseph, J., Sattenspiel, L., and Park, T. "Sexual Partner Selectiveness Effects of Homosexual HIV Transmission Dynamics." *Journal of Acquired Immune Deficiency Syndromes,* 1988, *1,* 486-504.

Lui, K.-J., Darrow, W. W., and Rutherford, G. W. III. "A Model-Based Estimate of the Mean Incubation Period for AIDS in Homosexual Men." *Science,* 1988, *240* (4857), 1333-1335.

May, R. M., and Anderson, R. M. "Transmission Dynamics of HIV Infection." *Nature,* 1987, *326,* 137-142.

May, R. M., and Anderson, R. M. "The Transmission Dynamics of Human Immunodeficiency Virus (HIV)." *Philosophical Transactions of the Royal Society,* 1988, B321, 565-607.

May, R. M., Anderson, R. M., and Blower, S. M. "The Epidemiology and Transmission Dynamics of HIV-AIDS." *Daedelus,* 1989, *118* (2), 163-201.

Medley, G. F., Anderson, R. M., Cox, D. R., and Billard, L. "Incubation Period of AIDS in Patients Infected via Blood Transfusion." *Nature,* 1987, *328,* 719-721.

Pickering, J., Wiley, J. A., Lieb, L. E., Walker, J., and Rutherford, G. W. "Modeling the Incidence of AIDS in New York, Los Angeles, and San Francisco." In J. C. Jager and E. J. Ruitenberg (eds.), *Statistical Analysis and Mathematical Modeling of AIDS.* Oxford, England: Oxford University Press, 1988.

Richardson, S. C., Caroni, C., and Papaevangelou, G. "Predicting the AIDS Epidemic from Trends Elsewhere." In J. C. Jager and E. J. Ruitenberg (eds.), *Statistical Analysis and Mathematical Modeling of AIDS.* Oxford, England: Oxford University Press, 1988.

Taylor, J.M.G. "Models for the HIV Infection and AIDS Epidemic in the United States." *Statistics in Medicine,* 1989, *8* (1), 45-58.

Wiley, J. A., Herschkorn, S. J., and Padian, N. S. "Heterogeneity in the Probability of HIV Transmission per Sexual Contact: The Case of Male-to-Female Transmission in Penile-Vaginal Intercourse." *Statistics in Medicine,* 1989, *8* (1), 93-102.

Edward H. Kaplan is associate professor of policy modeling and public management at the Yale School of Organization and Management and associate professor of operations research in Yale's Operations Research Department. He is an associate editor of the journals Operations Research *and* Journal of Sex Research *and chair of the College on Public Programs and Processes of the Institute for Management Sciences.*

In this chapter, the authors question current estimates of the AIDS incubation period drawn from convenience samples, citing potential difficulties with generalizability and selection bias.

Estimates of AIDS Incubation Periods from Convenience Samples

Paul R. Abramson, Richard A. Berk

The length of incubation, sometimes called the incubation period, is defined as "the period of time between exposure to a causative agent and the appearance of the first clinical manifestations of the disease" (Kelsey, Thompson, and Evans, 1986, p. 28). Length of incubation is a critical epidemiological parameter. Inferences about incubation affect descriptions of epidemic dynamics, estimates of the date of a common exposure, assessments of maximum infectiousness, and insights about the pathogenesis of disease (Sartwell, 1966). Estimates of incubation also have clinical significance. Advice to patients and their potential contacts obviously is influenced by assumptions about infectivity and variability in the incubation period (Bailey, 1975; Ho, Pomerantz, and Kaplan, 1988).

For human diseases, it is common for estimates of incubation length to be obtained from samples that are less than ideal. For example, data may be obtained only from people who seek treatment or who are properly diagnosed. Three questions naturally follow. First, one must consider the degree to which the estimates of incubation length may be generalized. For example, perhaps the people who seek treatment have especially virulent forms of the disease. Second, one must consider, in a similar fashion, whether estimates of the relationships between incubation length and other variables of interest, such as risk factors, may be generalized. For example, the importance of certain risk factors may be underestimated because the sample of people who seek treatment

---

Thanks go to Roderick J. A. Little and Howard Freeman for helpful suggestions on an earlier draft of this chapter.

are relatively homogeneous with respect to those risk factors. Finally, and more subtly, one must consider whether the sampling procedures produced an estimate of incubation period that statistically is unsound even for the population represented by the sample on hand. Sometimes this problem is called sample selection bias.

These questions carry over to recent research on AIDS, in which a number of investigators have attempted to estimate the incubation time for AIDS (Lui and others, 1986; Lui and Rutherford, 1988; Medley, Anderson, Cox, and Billard, 1987; Anderson, 1988). Relying primarily on patients infected through blood transfusions, Lui and his colleagues (1986) estimate the mean incubation time at 4.5 years, while in a subsequent study, with data drawn from a cohort of gay and bisexual men with hepatitis, Lui and Rutherford (1988) estimate the mean incubation time at 7.8 years (Lui and others, 1986; Lui and Rutherford, 1988). Similarly, Medley, Anderson, Cox, and Billard (1987), using blood transfusion data, estimate the mean incubation time at eight years. Such estimates are critical, in part because they represent inputs for estimates of the basic reproductive rate of AIDS (Kaplan, 1989a, 1989b; May and Anderson, 1987). The "reproductive rate" is the number of secondary infections per primary infection in a population of susceptibles.

In this chapter, we will summarize potential difficulties for both generalizability and selection bias when estimates of the length of incubation period for AIDS are obtained from convenience samples drawn from industrialized countries, such as a set of people who have had blood transfusions. The discussion of generalizability builds on common-sense notions of representativeness and, therefore, will be brief. Selection bias will be addressed in more depth, in part because some of the implications of convenience samples are counterintuitive. We stress at the outset, however, that our concerns are primarily substantive; our aim is to alert readers to the possible dangers of too readily accepting current estimates of the AIDS incubation period. Technical matters are kept to a minimum, with references provided to the relevant statistical literature. Finally, while we shall concentrate on blood transfusion samples used in research on the incubation period for AIDS, the issues raised apply to convenience samples of all kinds (such as individuals infected with hepatitis B).

External Validity with Convenience Samples

AIDS patients infected through blood transfusions clearly are not a probability sample of all persons with AIDS (Piot and others, 1988). Rather, when a group of such patients become subjects in a study of AIDS incubation periods, the result is a "convenience" sample whose relationships to one or more populations of interest are suspect.

Two kinds of generalizations must be considered. The first concerns inferences about univariate parameters from the sample to a specified population. Clearly, for example, one would be interested in estimates of the mean and median incubation period. (From a public policy perspective, there are a number of other parameter values one might like to estimate. For example, it could well be useful to estimate the proportion of persons with AIDS who are able to pay for their medical care, perhaps through a health insurance program at their place of work. However, these are not the concern of this chapter.)

Also of interest, however, might be estimates of the prevalence of AIDS infection cofactors. These estimates are critical because cofactors are relevant to both the transmission and pathogenesis of HIV infection and AIDS. For example, individuals who are particularly susceptible to AIDS often have chronically activated immune systems as a consequence of viral and parasitic antigenic exposure (Quinn and others, 1987). Similarly, sexually transmitted diseases, especially genital ulcer disease, increase susceptibility for HIV infection and AIDS (DeHovitz, 1986; Levy, 1988; Piot and others, 1987; World Health Organization, 1989a), while the herpesvirus, at least in the laboratory, acts on regulatory regions of HIV to enhance virus replication within the cell (Levy, 1988). Sexually transmitted diseases also appear to provoke a lymphocyte response that may increase virus inoculation from an HIV-infected individual or, conversely, may disrupt the integrity of the mucus or skin, which can facilitate the invasion of HIV into new hosts (DeHovitz, 1986). Finally, since research on retroviruses has suggested that infections tend to be "multiple-hit," phenomena and that a variety of cofactors are clearly relevant (for example, initial dose of the virus, age, and immunological status), the distribution of cofactors is especially important (Francis and Essex, 1978).

The second kind of generalization relates to multivariate inferences involving parameters to the joint distribution of particular variables. For example, one might simply want to estimate some bivariate measure of association, such as an odds ratio, between the length of the incubation period and a given cofactor. Alternatively, one might also want to estimate the full set of parameters of a Cox proportional hazard regression model with the length of incubation period as the outcome measure and a number of risk cofactors as "causal" variables. In the United States, relevant causal variables could include receptive anal intercourse (Kingsley and others, 1987), genital herpes (Levy, 1988), injection drug use (Kaplan, 1989a), antibodies to hepatitis B (Lui and Rutherford, 1988), and so forth. Similarly, in Central Africa, relevant causal variables could include injections from traditional medical practitioners (Quinn, Mann, Curran, and Piot, 1986), multiple viruses (such as hepatitis B or cytomegalovirus), multiple parasitic diseases (such as malaria, trypanosomiasis) (Marlik and Essex, 1987), sex with a prostitute, a history of prostitution, genital ulcers (Kreiss and others, 1986), and so forth.

It should be no surprise that estimates of both univariate and multivariate parameters, drawn from small convenience samples, may be terribly misleading if applied to the global population of AIDS patients. At present, there are at least 139,886 cases of AIDS worldwide, reported from 144 countries (World Health Organization, 1989b). This number, of course, is but a fraction of the millions of individuals presumed to be HIV infected (Quinn, Mann, Curran, and Piot, 1986). Thus, there is reason to suspect that small convenience samples, made up of individuals such as those who need blood transfusions in the United States, are not typical of either AIDS patients or HIV-infected individuals worldwide. Moreover, it seems reasonable to question whether characteristics of individuals in need of blood transfusions (such as being medically compromised) affect the length of the AIDS incubation period or the impact of potential HIV risk cofactors—given that seroconversion, infectivity, and incubation length are variable (Anderson and May, 1988; Levy, 1988; May, Anderson, and Blower, 1989).

However, it is one thing to observe that in principle convenience samples may not accurately represent a given population and another thing to demonstrate that substantively important differences exist. Yet data from transfusion samples themselves are unsettling. In particular, there is evidence that AIDS incubation periods are shorter for children and the elderly and much shorter for infants (May, Anderson, and Blower, 1989). If such variation exists within the transfusion samples, why not between transfusion samples and other samples? We stress, therefore, that while it is risky to generalize from studies of transfusion patients, we know of no compelling evidence on the direction and size of possible biases. In order to know those biases, one would have to have comparable sample data from other populations of interest, such as injection drug users. Such data are difficult to obtain.

Also, studies of transfusion patients from industrialized countries to date have been affected by "right-hand censoring." This effect occurs when the length of the study follow-up period is not long enough to observe the length of the incubation periods for all individuals who ultimately will contract AIDS. In other words, the sample from which estimates are made is limited to individuals who "convert" within the follow-up period. As a result, another kind of convenience sample is produced. This means, for example, that a study with a three-year follow-up cannot collect data on the fraction of the sample who contract AIDS more than three years after infection with HIV.

Clearly, such censoring will lead to underestimates in the length of the AIDS incubation period (Lawless, 1982; Lagakos, Barraj, and De Gruttola, 1988; De Gruttola and Lagakos, 1988). Such censoring also implies that the distribution of cofactors in people who convert quickly may not fairly represent the distribution of cofactors more generally and that estimates of any associations between cofactors and the length of the incubation periods are subject to the same concerns already described.

In short, estimates of the length of the AIDS incubation period from AIDS transfusion patients living in industrialized countries are affected by two kinds of nonprobability sampling mechanisms: the requirement that the HIV infection was contracted through a blood transfusion and the exclusion from the analysis of individuals whose incubation periods are longer than the period of time the study can stay in the field. Both mechanisms may seriously limit external validity. It is important to stress that similar problems may surface for any kind of sample not drawn by probability procedures.

Internal Validity with Convenience Samples

There are at least two occasions on which convenience samples may lead to data that are incomplete. First, for the population of interest, certain observations may be excluded. As Schneider (1986) points out, perhaps the most common instance occurs when measurement procedures restrict observations above some upper boundary or below some lower boundary. For example, current testing procedures for HIV antibodies may fail to detect antibody levels below some threshold. Or survey instruments that assess the number of sexual partners in the past year may inadvertently use ten as their highest category, when some unknown number of respondents have had more than ten partners. Thus, even if the entire population were studied, certain data points would be unavailable. Schneider (1986) calls this circumstance "truncation." (Truncation must be distinguished from population distributions that are naturally bounded, independent of how measures are collected. For example, the number of sexual partners is necessarily bounded from below at zero. While such distributions may create problems in conventional data analyses, truncation is not the cause.)

Truncation, which may be present before a sample is drawn, however, is not our concern. Instead, we are focusing on sampling procedures that result in some observations not being available above or below some boundary. For example, a sample of low-income people selected from an entire city's adult population obviously will not include any data on high-income individuals. Since selection for the sample was based on income, the observed income distribution, again using Schneider's (1986) language, is "censored."

There are many different definitions of truncation and censoring, depending in part on the academic tradition from which the literature draws (see, for example, Amemiya, 1985). At this point, we are restricting our attention to direct censoring on the particular variable of interest. There are also more complicated and subtle forms of censoring in which the censoring is indirect. For an accessible introduction to these issues, see Berk (1983).

Censoring may have important implications for the generalizability of any research and certainly of research on incubation times. However, censoring may also affect internal validity in ways that are somewhat counterintuitive. Consider the following example. The distribution of incubation periods is necessarily bounded at zero, probably peaks somewhere between two and four years, and almost certainly has a long tail. It may be reasonably described, therefore, by a log-normal distribution (Lawless, 1982), which by definition is normal once the logarithm is calculated.

In Figure 1, we show a hypothetical two-dimensional scatter plot in which the outcome variable (Y) is the logarithm of the incubation period (measured in months) and the explanatory variable (X) is the number of sexual partners per month—a relevant risk factor in Central Africa (Piot and others, 1988) and a critical variable in transmission probability (May, Anderson, and Blower, 1989). The 500 observations on the outcome variable were constructed from a fixed explanatory variable ranging from zero to ten, using a linear regression equation with an intercept of 4.0, a regression coefficient of -0.2, and a disturbance term drawn at random from a standard normal population. This model is simply the conventional linear regression model applied to a logged dependent variable (Lawless, 1982). Thus, the regression coefficient translates into a decline of 0.2 in the log of the incubation time for each additional sexual partner per month. In the original (not logged) units of incubation time, the regression coefficient represents a multiplicative factor of 0.82 for each additional sexual partner per month. In short, a greater number of partners is associated with a shorter incubation period.

Given how the data were constructed, the first column in Table 1 holds no surprises. The sample estimates for the bivariate regression of the outcome variable on the explanatory variable are all close to the known population parameters; the estimates for the intercept and slope are 4.01 and -0.20 respectively. Thus, the regression line shown in Figure 1 looks just about the way it should.

The story is quite different under censoring. As a demonstration of "direct" or "explicit" censoring, all observations with values on the outcome variable of greater than 3.0 were deleted. In other words, 3.0 serves as a threshold below which the observation for the log of incubation period must fall if these values and associated values of the explanatory variable are to be included in the sample. Such censoring might occur in practice if data on a cohort of blood transfusion patients, who received their infected transfusions during the same month, were followed for only twenty months.

Figure 2 shows the results. It is immediately apparent that compared to Figure 1, the scatter plot has been shifted downward and to the right. Thus, Table 1 shows that for the censored data, the mean of X has increased and the mean of Y decreased. In addition, the variability of X and Y have both been reduced. (Since censoring in our example requires deleting certain values of Y and X's with which they are linked—"listwise"

Figure 1. Uncensored Data

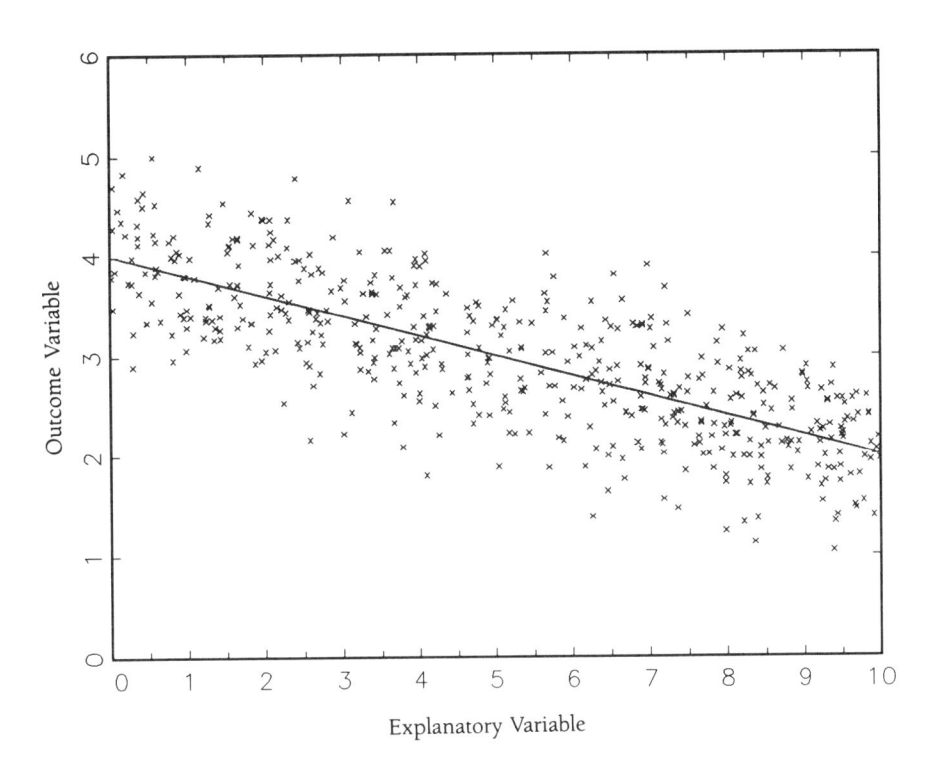

Table 1. Statistics for Uncensored and Censored Samples

	Uncensored	Censored
Mean X	5.15	7.12
Mean Y	2.97	2.36
Standard deviation X	2.91	2.07
Standard deviation Y	0.76	0.43
Intercept	4.01	3.02
Slope	−0.20	−0.9
N	500	257

Figure 2. Censored Data

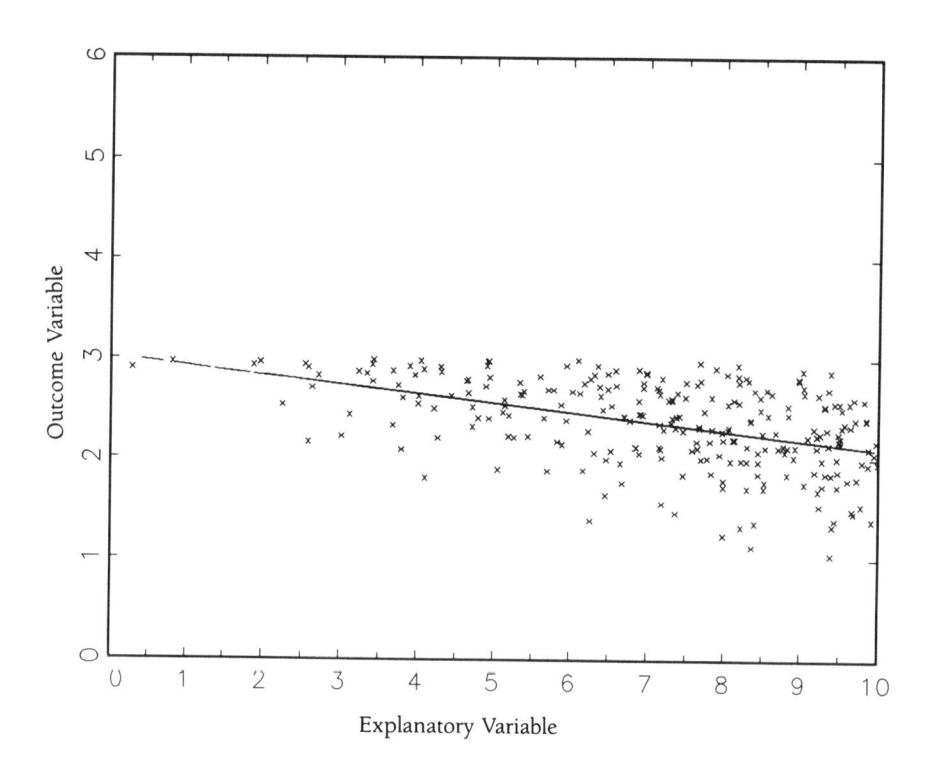

[Scatter plot with Outcome Variable (0-6) on y-axis and Explanatory Variable (0-10) on x-axis, showing a downward-sloping regression line through data points concentrated below y=3.]

deletion—censoring affects entire cases. In addition, while the censoring was done through a threshold on Y, the negative association between X and Y, by construction, means that deleting large values of Y tends—but *only* tends—to delete small values of X.) These changes go directly to the question of external validity already discussed. In other words, censoring affects not just estimates for the variable being censored but for all variables associated with it.

Figure 2 also reveals that the top of the scatter plot has been flattened. When the regression line is fitted to the censored data, a less steep slope is produced. Looking again at Table 1, the slope is changed from -0.20 to -0.09, a drop of about 50 percent in absolute value. The intercept also is dramatically altered, although the intercept is typically a less interesting parameter. In short, censoring through a threshold on incubation period attenuates the bivariate relationship observed between incubation period and the number of sexual partners. This is always true more generally, whether the threshold on the outcome variable is from above or from below and in the bivariate or multivariate case (Goldberger, 1981). This general issue also speaks to external validity, and one may legitimately ask whether the estimated regression line, at least in some sense, is appropriate for the censored sample.

Unfortunately, the answer is no. To begin, the sample is of little interest in itself. The point is to learn things from the sample that may be generalized beyond the data at hand. In that case, what is the appropriate population? We already have illustrated how generalizations to the original population are misleading. Alternatively, suppose one defined the relevant population as all possible samples that would have been produced by sampling procedures identical to those we employed in our illustration; that is, our data are one possible realization of a data-generating process, which includes the censoring mechanism. Similar rationales are routinely used in all sorts of applications, especially when random sampling from some known population is impossible (Barnett, 1982). For instance, our earlier example of low-income adults could be viewed as one realization of a large number of samples of low-income adults, each selected through the same censoring procedure.

Yet this strategy fails as well. A close look at Figure 2 suggests that as one moves from right to left, there is a decreasing tendency for the observations to fall above the regression line. This pattern implies that the linear form is incorrect. In fact, the censoring has necessarily altered the data so that the assumed (and built-in) linear relationship no longer holds (Berk, 1983). As a result, the residuals and the explanatory variable will tend to be positively associated; as the explanatory variable increases, the balance of residuals will become more positive. Any association between an explanatory variable and the disturbances, in turn, is well known to bias estimates of the slope, even for a population as redefined here. Put another way, the linear regression estimates of the intercept and slope neglect the mechanism by which the censoring occurred and therefore fail to represent properly the processes generating the data. As a result, the censoring process and the relationship between the outcome and explanatory variables are confounded. In fact, because the least squares regression line fits the data as given, no such association exists; that is, the association is already incorporated incorrectly into the regression estimates. The point is that with this confounding of the role of the explanatory variable with the role of the disturbances, effects attributed to the explanatory variable in part belong to the disturbances. Readers interested in a more formal explanation of the problem should consult Lawless (1982) where it becomes apparent that the usual likelihood function for the regression model with normally distributed disturbances leaves out an important piece.

Figures 1 and 2 illustrate "explicit selection" (Goldberger, 1981). They also illustrate "endogenous sampling" (Amemiya, 1985). The basic problem is that cases are selected via an explicit threshold on the outcome (endogenous) variable, resulting in confounding of the selection process with the substantive process under study. In particular, under explicit selection, all regression coefficients are attenuated (Goldberger, 1981). This is related to sampling procedures commonly used in retrospective case-control studies. In such studies, data on some arbitrary number of cases and some arbitrary number of controls are collected (for example, 200 of each). The "cases" may be individuals with cancer and the "controls" may be individuals who are cancer free. In effect, one is sampling on the outcome variable in a nonrepresentative manner. However, since the outcome is nominal, certain kinds of relationships may be estimated in an unbiased manner. For instance, the "odds multiplier" may be properly estimated with logistic regression (Holland and Rubin, 1988).

There are many other kinds of censoring. In particular, a sample may be selected through a variable that is neither an outcome variable nor an explanatory variable for the relationship of interest. Returning to the use of transfusion patients in studies on the AIDS incubation period, potential subjects are chosen because of the way they became infected with HIV. Such censoring is often called "incidental" (Heckman, 1979; Goldberger, 1981; Berk, 1983) because the selection is not based directly on the outcome variable but on some other variable.

Whether incidental censoring leads to the sorts of biases already described depends on whether the outcome variable (such as incubation time) and the censoring variable (such as receiving a blood transfusion) are statistically related after the impact of the explanatory variables is taken into account (Heckman, 1979; Berk, 1983). In other words, the critical question is whether the partial correlation between the outcome variable and the censoring variable is zero, holding constant all of the explanatory variables. (There are other assumptions that need to be made, such as no measurement error in the explanatory variables, but these assumptions are not essential to the points being made about censoring.) The partial correlation will not be zero when variables affecting both the outcome variable and selection variable are not among the set of explanatory variables. In the case of transfusion patients in industrialized countries and the AIDS incubation period, a host of health-related candidates come to mind (such as the magnitude of HIV inoculation, diet, occupation). When the partial correlation is not zero, internal validity will be in doubt. And the estimates may be systematically too low or systematically too high. (While sampling on the outcome variable is always risky, sampling on explanatory variables will typically be sound. Stratified probability sampling, for example, fixes the proportions of cases to be sampled across different categories, or levels, on one or more explanatory variables and then samples randomly within strata. For example, in a study of incubation periods, one might stratify by age and oversample the very young and very old.)

Over the past several decades, a number of statistical procedures have been devised that, in the face of censoring and under some circumstances, produce unbiased or at least consistent estimates of key parameters. Reviews of such techniques can now be found in a number of texts (Lawless, 1982; Amemiya, 1985; Schneider, 1986). While the details are well beyond the scope of this chapter, all rest on an ability to represent the selection process in a formal statistical model. Suffice it to say, there is considerable controversy about the degree to which the essentials of that process can be captured effectively (Manski, 1989).

Conclusion

In summary, it is probably fair to say that all empirical research on incubation periods rests on censored samples and that as a result more than external validity is in jeopardy. Any attempt to link explanatory variables, such as risk factors, to the length of incubation periods invites serious bias. At the least, these biases need to be acknowledged. In addition, however, effort should be made to apply existing statistical technology that might improve matters (Brookmeyer and Gail, 1988; Lagakos, Barraj, and De Gruttola, 1988). Ideally, data should be collected so that censoring is unlikely to occur; probability samples should be taken with cases followed prospectively. Finally, it is critical to stress again that knowledge of incubation periods of HIV is sorely inadequate. As a result, facts about infectivity (Ho, Pomerantz, and Kaplan, 1988) and about the ultimate proliferation of HIV (Abramson, 1988; Abramson and Rothschild, 1988; Isham, 1988; Curran and others, 1988; Dietz and Hadeler, 1988; May and Anderson, 1987) remain largely unknown.

References

Abramson, P. R. "Sexual Assessment and the Epidemiology of AIDS." *Journal of Sex Research,* 1988, *25* (3), 323-346.

Abramson, P. R., and Rothschild, B. "Sex, Drugs, and Matrices: Mathematical Prediction of HIV Infection." *Journal of Sex Research,* 1988, *25* (1), 106-122.

Amemiya, T. *Advanced Econometrics.* Cambridge, England: Cambridge University Press, 1985.

Anderson, R. M. "The Epidemiology of HIV Infection: Variable Incubation Plus Infectious Periods and Heterogeneity in Sexual Activity." *Journal of the Royal Statistical Society,* 1988, Series A, *151,* Part 1, 66-93.

Anderson, R. M., and May, R. M. "Epidemiological Parameters of HIV Transmission." *Nature,* 1988, *333,* 514-519.

Bailey, N.T.J. *The Mathematical Theory of Infectious Diseases.* London: Griffin, 1975.

Barnett, V. *Comparative Statistical Inference.* New York: Wiley, 1982.

Berk, R. A. "An Introduction to Sample Selection Bias in Sociological Data." *American Sociological Review,* 1983, *48,* 386-398.

Brookmeyer, R., and Gail, M. H. "A Method for Obtaining Short-Term Projections and Lower Bounds on the Size of the AIDS Epidemic." *Journal of the American Statistical Association,* 1988, *83* (402), 301-308.

Curran, J. W., Jaffe, H. W., Hardy, A. M., Morgan, W. M., Selik, R. M., and Dondero,

T. J. "Epidemiology of HIV Infection and AIDS in the United States." *Science,* 1988, *239,* 610-616.

De Gruttola, V., and Lagakos, S. W. *Analysis of Doubly Censored Survival Data with Applications to AIDS.* Unpublished paper. Cambridge, Mass.: Department of Biostatistics, Harvard University, 1988.

DeHovitz, J. A. "A Perspective on the Heterosexual Transmission of the Acquired Immunodeficiency Syndrome." *New York State Journal of Medicine,* 1986, *86,* 117-118.

Dietz, K., and Hadeler, K. P. "Epidemiological Models for Sexually Transmitted Diseases." *Journal of Mathematical Biology,* 1988, *26,* 1-25.

Francis, D. P., and Essex, M. "Leukemia and Lymphoma: Infrequent Manifestations of Common Viral Infection? A Review." *Journal of Infectious Disease,* 1978, *138,* 916-923.

Goldberger, A. S. "Linear Regression After Selection." *Journal of Econometrics,* 1981, *15,* 357-366.

Heckman, J. J. "Sample Selection Bias as a Specification Error." *Econometrics,* 1979, *45,* 153-161.

Ho, D. D., Pomerantz, R. J., and Kaplan, J. C. "Pathogenesis of Infection with Human Immunodeficiency Virus." *New England Journal of Medicine,* 1988, *317,* 278-286.

Holland, P. W., and Rubin, D. B. "Causal Inference in Retrospective Studies." *Evaluation Review,* 1988, *12,* 203-231.

Isham, V. "Mathematical Modeling of the Transmission Dynamics of HIV Interaction and AIDS: A Review." *Journal of the Royal Statistical Society,* 1988, Series A, Part 1, *151* (1), 5-30.

Kaplan, E. H. "Needles That Kill: Modeling Human Immunodeficiency Virus Transmission via Shared Drug Injection Equipment in Shooting Galleries." *Reviews of Infectious Diseases,* 1989a, *11* (2), 289-298.

Kaplan, E. H. "What Are the Risks of Risky Sex? Modeling the AIDS Epidemic." *Operations Research,* 1989b, *37,* 198-209.

Kelsey, J. L., Thompson, W. D., and Evans, A. S. *Methods in Observational Epidemiology.* New York: Oxford University Press, 1986.

Kingsley, L. A., Kaslow, R., Rinaldo, C. R., Detre, K., Odaka, N., VanRaden, M., Detels, R., Polk, B. F., Chmiel, J., Kelsey, S. F., Ostrow, D., and Visscher, B. "Risk Factors for Seroconversion to Human Immunodeficiency Virus Among Male Homosexuals." *Lancet,* 1987, (8529), 345-348.

Kreiss, J. K., Koech, D., Plummer, F. A., Holmes, K. K., Lightfoote, M., Piot, P., Ronald, A. R., Ndinya-achola, J. O., D'Costa, L. J., Roberts, P., Ngugi, E. N., and Quinn, T. C. "AIDS Virus Infection in Nairobi Prostitutes." *New England Journal of Medicine,* 1986, *314,* 414-418.

Lagakos, S. W., Barraj, L. M., and De Gruttola, V. *Nonparametric Analysis of Truncated Survival Data with Application to AIDS.* Unpublished paper. Cambridge, Mass.: Department of Biostatistics, Harvard University, 1988.

Lawless, J. F. *Statistical Models and Methods for Lifetime Data.* New York: Wiley, 1982.

Levy, J. A. "Mysteries of HIV: Challenges for Therapy and Prevention." *Nature,* 1988, *333,* 519-522.

Lui, K., Lawrence, D. N., Morgan, W. M., Peterman, T. A., Haverkos, H. W., and Bregman, D. J. "A Model-Based Approach for Estimating the Mean Incubation Period of Transfusion-Associated Acquired Immunodeficiency Syndrome." *Proceedings of the National Academy of Sciences,* 1986, *83,* 3051-3055.

Lui, K.-J., and Rutherford, G. W. III. "A Model-Based Estimate of the Mean Incubation Period for AIDS in Homosexual Men." *Science,* 1988, *240* (4857), 1333-1335.

Manski, C. F. "Anatomy of the Selection Problem." *Journal of Human Resources*, 1989, 24 (3), 343-360.
Marlik, R. G., and Essex, M. "Africa and the Biology of Human Immunodeficiency Virus." *Journal of the American Medical Association*, 1987, 257, 2632-2633.
May, R. M., and Anderson, R. M. "Transmission Dynamics of HIV Infection." *Nature*, 1987, 326, 137-142.
May, R. M., Anderson, R. M., and Blower, S. M. "The Epidemiology and Transmission Dynamics of HIV-AIDS." *Daedalus*, 1989, 118 (2), 163-201.
Medley, G. F., Anderson, R. M., Cox, D. R., and Billard, L. "Incubation Period of AIDS in Patients Infected via Blood Transfusion." *Nature*, 1987, 328, 719-721.
Piot, P., Kreiss, J. D., Jackonia, O. N., Ngugi, E. N., Simoneson, J. N., Cameron, D. W., Taelman, H., and Plummer, F. A. "Heterosexual Transmission of HIV." *AIDS*, 1987, 1, 199-206.
Piot, P., Plummer, F. A., Mhalu, F. S., Lamboray, J., Chin, J., and Mann, J. M. "AIDS: An International Perspective." *Science*, 1988, 239, 573-579.
Quinn, T. C., Mann, J. M., Curran, J. W., and Piot, P. "AIDS in Africa: An Epidemiologic Paradigm." *Science*, 1986, 234, 955-963.
Quinn, T. C., Piot, P., McCormick, J. B., Feinsod, F. M., Taelman, H., Kapita, B., Stevens, W., and Fauci, A. S. "Serologic and Immunologic Studies in Patients with AIDS in North America and Africa." *Journal of the American Medical Association*, 1987, 257, 2617-2621.
Sartwell, P. E. "The Incubation Period and the Dynamics of Infectious Disease." *American Journal of Epidemiology*, 1966, 83, 204-216.
Schneider, H. *Truncated and Censored Samples from Normal Populations.* New York: Marcel Dekker, 1986.
World Health Organization. "Sexually Transmitted Diseases as a Risk Factor for HIV Transmission." *Journal of Sex Research*, 1989a, 26, 272-275.
World Health Organization. *Update: AIDS Cases.* Geneva, Switzerland: World Health Organization, 1989b.

Paul R. Abramson is associate professor of psychology at the University of California, Los Angeles (UCLA), editor of the Journal of Sex Research, *and technical adviser to the World Health Organization Global Program on AIDS.*

Richard A. Berk is a professor in the Department of Sociology and Program in Social Statistics at UCLA. He is vice-chair of the board of directors of the Social Science Research Council and former chair of the Methodology Section of the American Sociological Association.

Ethnographic methods complement standard treatment or control group studies by providing contextual and culturally sensitive information to administrators and service providers in AIDS prevention programs.

Ethnographic Evaluation of AIDS Prevention Programs: Better Data for Better Programs

Jean J. Schensul, Stephen L. Schensul

Early in the AIDS epidemic, evaluators and intervention researchers recognized that experimental design and other traditional approaches to research and evaluation could not provide sufficient information to program developers and policy makers to guide interventions in communities. Over the past five years, ethnography has demonstrated its utility in collecting qualitative and quantitative planning data on the life-styles, social networks, needle-sharing activities, sexual patterns, and decision-making processes of IV drug users, their partners, and prostitutes (Downing, 1988; Feldman and Johnson, 1986; Page, 1988; Sterk, 1988). The focus of this chapter is on the use of ethnography as a tool in monitoring and evaluating AIDS prevention programs.

AIDS is a disease that challenges all social science researchers to identify valid and reliable methods of investigation leading to a better understanding of high-risk behavior and its prevention. The challenges lie in obtaining accurate descriptions of risk behavior, in locating and identifying those at risk, in developing appropriate interventions, and in accurately assessing behavioral change. The identification of individuals at risk is problematic because those most at risk for AIDS are also most likely to experience discrimination resulting from their IV drug use, sexual preference, or ethnic identity. Thus, they may prefer to remain unidentified or to respond inaccurately to survey and self-report methods of data collection. The measurement of change in risk behavior is difficult because, unlike the behaviors that lead to transmission of other diseases, the exchanges that result in the transmission of HIV are private and not readily observable. New methods for observing the social context of needle use and sharing and of sexual activity must be found in order to guide more effective interventions and to determine behavioral changes.

This chapter will describe an alternative, ethnographic approach to research that holds promise for understanding the ways in which communities are responding to AIDS and the degree to which intervention strategies now in use are effective. The chapter will discuss current informational needs in AIDS prevention programs, examine the interplay of ethnography and evaluation, and describe steps in ethnographic evaluation of AIDS programs useful for program planners and evaluators.

Gaps in AIDS-Related Research

AIDS presents a number of unique features that create difficulties for research and intervention. The mystery and fear surrounding the disease have been complicating factors in the development of effective intervention programs. Because etiology and modes of transmission only recently have been clearly identified (Flam and Stein, 1986), myths and misunderstandings about AIDS and its transmission are widespread (AIDS Community Research Group, 1988, 1989; DiClemente, Boyer, and Morales, 1988; Estrada, DeBoor, Fernandez, and Dalgorn, 1988). These confusions have led to a variety of interpretations of AIDS and its etiology and to different community and individual responses to the disease (Hispanic Health Alliance, 1988). These cultural differences are not well understood, and existing interventions do little to explore them or to take them into serious consideration (Peterson and Morin, 1988). The available quantitative measures of AIDS intervention outcomes do not adequately describe inter- and intrapopulation variation before or during an intervention, nor do they examine the relationship between such variations and patterned differences in outcomes.

Further, AIDS is associated with behavior that is considered taboo, illegal, or immoral. Individuals involved in exchanging sex for money or drugs, using drugs intravenously, or engaging in oral or anal sex without protection of condoms (especially with partners of the same gender) often feel that these behaviors should be kept confidential or that they are unsafe if they reveal their involvement. Those people most at risk for exposure to the virus may be the least attracted to research or interventions intended to protect them.

Finally, even the general effectiveness of the now widespread efforts to stop the transmission of the disease is as yet undetermined (Antoniskis, Sattler, and Leedom, 1988; Mason and others, 1988; Hopkins, 1987). Available means of prevention are limited to needle cleaning and the use of condoms, behaviors that are difficult to sustain and even more difficult to measure. In both cases, compliance is unlikely because a conscious decision must be made to use these methods at all times, especially on occasions usually associated with spontaneity, compulsivity, and the casting aside of control (Richwald, Schneider-Monoz, and Valdez, 1989; Feldblum and Fortney, 1988). Additionally, in the case of condoms, the partner's consent is required.

Despite these limitations, studies on the current status of AIDS knowledge and behavior indicate that both the general population and those participating in high-risk behavior have increased their knowledge of modes of AIDS transmission and ways of preventing exposure to HIV (Becker and Joseph, 1988; Fineberg, 1988; Fischl, 1988). These results, however, are inconclusive, inconsistent, and based on self-reported responses to quantitative survey instruments. Little has been done to validate or explicate these results with other research methods. As a result, we do not know to what extent reported behavioral changes can be attributed to interventions or to other factors. Nor do we know the differential effects of these changes on target populations. In addition, there are many unanswered questions about the effects of knowledge of seropositivity on behavior, about the relationship between increased knowledge of AIDS prevention and behavior change (Selwyn and others, 1987), and about what most effectively brings about behavioral change in those engaged in high-risk behavior.

The Need for Ethnographic Research on AIDS-Related Behavior

The lack of satisfactory answers to such questions has led some health science researchers to propose ethnography as a critical aspect of evaluation research. The discovery methods of ethnography or ethnographic evaluation may be cited as one solution to health policy, service delivery, or program evaluation problems under the following circumstances:

1. The disease is new and its natural history and social definition are relatively unknown or emerging. Although the transmission of HIV through the exchange of infected blood and semen are the most common means of transmission of AIDS among heterosexual black, Hispanic, Southeast Asian, and American Indian communities, these populations are culturally differentiated and intraculturally diverse. Interpretations of disease, risk, and risk prevention differ.

2. The target population is new, unknown, unpopular, or difficult to reach by public health officials, physicians, and other professionals. AIDS has had a disproportionate effect on those who are socially, economically, and politically marginal (gay and bisexual men, poor African American and Latino men, and their sex partners) and on those who are viewed by public health officials as hard-to-reach populations.

3. Existing research paradigms (such as survey research, experimental

and quasi-experimental designs, and epidemiology) do not provide satisfactory answers to questions or problems concerning the environment in which the disease is spread, the vectors or vehicles for its contagion, popular responses to the problem, or unexplained differential or unanticipated effects of the disease or the public response to it.

4. Existing interventions have not solved the problem of infection or transmission. This is the case for malaria (Sevilla-Casa, 1989), diarrhea, and acute respiratory infection, as well as AIDS.

These considerations have persuaded such institutions as the World Health Organization, the National Institute on Drug Abuse, and the Centers for Disease Control to promote the use of ethnographic methods in AIDs research and evaluation. Both the history and methods of anthropology support this choice.

Anthropologists are best known for ethnographic research. The history of anthropology is associated with descriptions of exotic, remote, and culturally different people and environments. Anthropologists are well recognized as sympathetic to the interests of politically, socially, culturally, and economically marginal communities (Barger and Reza, 1987; Schensul and Schensul, 1978; Stull, Grell, and Weston, 1985) and have engaged in long-term field research in such communities throughout the world. Anthropology as a discipline has placed strong value on sound and rigorous research in these environments (Pelto and Pelto, 1978; Bernard, 1988).

Ethnography offers methods to identify, observe, document, and analyze culture (patterned beliefs and behaviors) in communities, institutions, and target populations under difficult field circumstances. In addition, the ethnographic perspective insists on identification and interpretation of the meanings behind observed behaviors, such as responses to disease (Werner and Schoepfle, 1987a, 1987b; Weller and Romney, 1988).

Ethnographers assume that patterns of behavior and their interpretation vary with ethnicity or cultural identity and, further, that ethnic groups are characterized by intraethnic diversity that must always be taken into consideration. Ethnographic methods are generally utilized to understand how and why systems function, in what ways people interact with them, and how they interpret and explain both the systems and their own interactions with them. In AIDS programming, the behaviors and ways of thinking of newly affected target populations are relatively unknown to health policy makers. When these populations do not respond to interventions or services in expected ways, ethnography can offer new interpretations to health decision makers and members of the target population themselves.

Ethnographic methods are eclectic. Anthropologists and other ethnographers usually "triangulate" a combination of qualitative and quantitative methods to obtain comprehensive program descriptions (Fetterman, 1984; LeCompte and Goetz, 1984; Center for New Schools, 1976). Qualitative methods of investigation include the use of observation, interviewing, program documentation, and logs or diaries. These methods have been discussed in the literature extensively (Pelto and Pelto, 1978; Bernard, 1988) and will not be described in detail here.

Qualitative methods are used for two major purposes: first, to construct a systematic description of the way in which a community, service delivery program, set of activities, or other social system works; and, second, to identify or discover critical factors that account for the difference in the patterns of interaction of individuals with that system. For example, typical questions about intravenous drug use for an outreach demonstration project in Hartford, Connecticut, call for qualitative methods of investigation and include the following (Institute for Community Research, 1989): What is the pattern of drug distribution in X neighborhood? What differences are there among addicts who live in and use X neighborhood? How do these differences come into play on the street in terms of different patterns of obtaining and using different types of drugs? These are questions that are difficult, if not impossible, to answer with survey techniques. They are also questions that involve a relatively large unit of analysis, such as a section of a city or a special population.

What Is Ethnographic Evaluation?

The term *ethnographic evaluation* represents a contradiction for the following reason. Evaluation refers to judgments against an already defined standard; ethnography constructs a theory to account for or to predict the ways in which cultural systems function. Evaluation is prescriptive; ethnography is descriptive (Wolcott, 1984). However, the two approaches can interface. Effective evaluation tests outcomes against a theory of action; thus, it presupposes a clear theoretical framework, clearly articulated goals and objectives, and an action plan (Rossi and Freeman, 1989; Suchman, 1967). Ethnography is a set of "discovery procedures" through which theory of action—or program theory—is generated and goals, objectives, and action can be defined clearly as they are implemented.

Ethnography is most useful when theory, standards, goals, and objectives are viewed as "fuzzy," flexible, discoverable, and changeable—in other words, when it can assist in generating or discovering the theory and methods underlying a program approach. Ethnography works best in evaluation when the model is emerging in the early stages of program development or when the program is viewed as constantly adapting to changing circumstances.

Evaluation, especially those approaches utilizing experimental or quasi-experimental designs and quantitative outcome measures, assumes clear-cut positive or negative outcomes with a finite number of outcome measures. Ethnography works well when there is a stated design to seek expanded and unanticipated outcomes, accept and explore negative outcomes, and recognize that the target population is diverse and unknown and that the program is likely to affect that population is different and not fully predictable ways. Quantitative evaluation of individual outcomes generally compares "classes" of individuals; ethnography is most useful in examining and explaining differential outcomes and variation in outcomes among individuals or across subgroups within the target population.

Sequence of Steps in Ethnographic Program Evaluation

Entering the Program. Ethnographic evaluators can be utilized best if they begin by looking at the conceptualization of the program and if their research is integrated with the day-to-day activities of the program. Entry involves discovering the theoretical framework of the program, defining goals and objectives with program staff, understanding the structure of the program, observing interventions, developing ways of describing program activities, assessing behavioral and knowledge change in the participants, and organizing appropriate feedback sessions.

These programs may have multiple target groups and staffs and be differentiated by ethnicity, gender, HIV status, education, and other factors. They may provide services in multiple sites. In addition, they are susceptible to changes in administration and staff, funding level, organizational and national policies, competition from other programs in the environment, the results of new research, and many other factors that may affect program implementation and outcomes.

It is helpful to think of AIDS programs as including a context (political, social, economic, cultural, and physical setting), an organizational base, a target population, a program standard (theoretical framework, goals, objectives, and action plan), inputs or resources, process, and consequences and outcomes. A comprehensive evaluation must take all of these program elements and their interactive effects into consideration. Process and outcomes may or may not be anticipated, intended, expected, or recognized, and the ethnographer may be in a unique position to detect them.

Establishing the Conceptual Model of the Program. The next step in ethnographic evaluation is to develop with program staff the perceived operating hypotheses underlying the program. The theory of the program may or may not be well articulated. The conceptual model consists of dependent variables and independent variables.

Dependent variables include measures of health status, health knowledge or behavior, and health care use. These variables, once defined, can be translated into problem statements. The problem statement can then be phrased in terms of the desired outcome. For example, in most AIDS prevention programs targeted to men and women involved in injection drug use, the dependent variable is the degree of exposure to HIV or the risk for transmitting HIV. The problem can be defined as the number of injection drug users (IDUs) engaged in high-risk behavior or as the desired outcome, a reduction in risk behavior among adult IDUs.

Independent variables include the factors believed to affect the problem. They may include the need for income (as in the exchange of sex for money), the degree of information available about risk behaviors and how to prevent them, the degree of family support for those at risk, addiction, the availability of treatment programs, the perceived effects of bleach on works, the cost of clean needles, the availability and cost of high-quality condoms, beliefs about condom use, as well as many other factors. Each of these variables can be phrased as a problem to be corrected that may then affect the status of the dependent variables, thus influencing outcomes.

One of the major problems in any evaluation task is that program personnel do not necessarily translate program activities into an evaluation model, and they may not be able to define independent and dependent variables. Ethnographic evaluation can assist them through staff interviews and field research on the target population. In addition, field research can determine whether the independent variables are central to the problem.

Setting Goals and Objectives. Those factors considered modifiable in the program model should be identified with specific program goals and objectives. Program goals and objectives should represent a clear, action-oriented operationalization of these independent variables. This framework is a critical element in guiding the evaluation process. Program staff who choose addiction as the most significant independent variable will organize prevention programs around reduction of addiction through treatment programs. Program staff who identify the cost of clean needles as the primary factor will not be able to develop intervention programs based on their interpretation since in most cases, the distribution of needles is prohibited. They may choose other factors, however, such as condom use, bleach distribution, and street education focusing on condom use.

Developing an Effective and Ongoing Research Design. Developing an effective and ongoing evaluation design requires integration of the program design and the evaluation design. In this way, program staff will understand the purpose of the evaluation, the reasons for data collection, and ways of using the information to improve their performance and outcomes. A "close fit" avoids the problem of evaluating the program from the single perspective of either the evaluator or the program staff.

The matter of how to organize ethnographic evaluation research in AIDS intervention and prevention programs involves both structural and staffing decisions. In our opinion, the most effective structure for carrying out ethnographic evaluation is to give anthropologists both internal and external evaluation roles. In this arrangement, program staff are working together with anthropologists to conceptualize, design, and carry out data collection procedures. Both the internal team (program staff) and the anthropologists as external evaluators analyze the data. In this way, program staff can define the direct benefits of the evaluation to them, are less likely to be threatened, more likely to accept and even to shape feedback, and more likely to be able to improve their own evaluations in the future. To be effective, however, the external ethnographers must participate in the documentation process along with program staff.

Ethnographic evaluation should be explained and integrated at all levels of the project and should be considered the responsibility of all project staff, rather than that of the outside ethnographer alone. We do not recommend differentiating and isolating the ethnographic evaluator's role from other activities in the project. While the information collected may be accurate and comprehensive, separation creates a structure in which the information is not easily integrated into the activities of the program. In addition, the ethnographer's questions and observations may be seen as intrusive and threatening. Ethnographers have often reported isolation, frustration, marginality, and unclear role definition.

Developing Appropriate Methods for Collecting Qualitative and Quantitative Data. Methods involving program staff should be culturally appropriate, cost effective, simple to use, integrated into service delivery, and organized to provide regular feedback to program staff. Methods involving ethnographers should be unobtrusive and should be organized to provide regular, organized, formal, and informal feedback. For example, outreach workers should not be expected to turn in elaborate field notes on a daily basis, but each week they might be assigned one specific question for investigation on the street, such as "Why are injection drug users reluctant to bring their sex partners or spouses to the program?" or "Where are the neighborhood locations where young men exchange sex for drugs, and how are these locations used?" Social workers should not be expected to fill in elaborate descriptions of clients for their case records, but they can be asked to participate in the development of a client encounter form that includes all the information they and the evaluators believe is important to assess the utility of an intervention.

The involvement of program staff in data collection is subject to the following limitations:

1. Program staff cannot act and observe themselves at the same time. This appears obvious; however, program staff are often expected to describe and document their intervention activities. They can only be expected to describe the sequence of their actions and the way in which individuals or groups responded in general terms. The fine detail or "thick description" that is obtained through observation is lost to the actor. The subtle effects of interventions or new information about risk behavior, use of language, and cultural concepts can only be identified by someone in an observer role.

2. Program staff or outreach workers are not trained to do ethnographic observations or in-depth interviewing. While they may be highly

knowledgeable, they must be trained to observe systematically and without bias. While they may have experience writing client case histories, these case materials are usually written in "shorthand" to address the informational needs of a service provider. They are likely to be inconsistent, problem focused, and, from the point of view of research, incomplete. Even when trained, not all program administrators or service providers enjoy the rigor of observing, interviewing, and recording, nor do they see the value of such activities to the program. Street outreach workers usually have limited time with program participants and are pressed to identify enough clients to meet program needs.

In our experience, a number of strategies can be used to address these problems. First, program staff should be hired only if they have some appreciation for information collection as a part of their work. The integration of evaluation research and service can only be successful if program staff are not resistant to the systematic recording of information on program participants, activities, and contexts.

Second, program staff and trained ethnographers can work in teams. The ethnographer acts as documenter, the program staff as informants. Both participate in the program. This arrangement avoids the expectation that program staff will keep field notes or systematic logs, but it permits staff to participate in the formation and analysis of these notes and logs.

Third, program staff can be asked to collect qualitative or quantitative information around specific issues. For example, staff of Hartford's three-year NIDA outreach demonstration project, Project COPE (Community Outreach Prevention Effort), collected observational information on patterns of street activity for ten to twenty minutes each hour on target days of the week. They asked targeted questions to potential participants about reasons why sex partners are not referred to the program, and they sought out participant "dropouts" on the street to discover their reasons for avoiding a program component. Next staff were asked to pursue reasons why injection drug users believed that alcohol pads could be substituted for bleach in preventing contact with HIV.

Program staff and outreach workers can be trained to carry out effective observations, interviewing, and systematic qualitative and quantitative data collection. However, the collection of useful qualitative data requires a considerable amount of time because the quality of the data depends on the level of knowledge, interpretation, and curiosity of the interviewer. Good qualitative interviewing requires a theoretical perspective, deepening knowledge of the topic, and good interactive skills, along with the ability to ask, probe, record, analyze in the interview, and continue to question until the topic is logically exhausted. While quantitative data can be routinely collected by staff who understand the issues and the instrument, both time and extensive training are needed for staff to develop qualitative data and question frames, to write, and to review.

Conclusion

Traditional anthropological ethnography and fieldwork was designed in the context of long-term, intensive participant observation in non-Western cultures. In the last three decades, the methodology has been applied to rural and urban communities in both the developed and the developing world, as well as to nonresidential contexts such as political, religious, and medical institutions. Its involvement in the evaluation process is even more recent, beginning with evaluation of educational programs in the 1970s (Fetterman, 1984) and including its utilization in operations research and "rapid assessment" (Scrimshaw and Hurtado, 1988). Ethnographic methods most often have been called into play as a result of the unexplained failure or lack of acceptance of programs such as oral rehydration therapy (for life-threatening diarrhea in the Third World), childhood immunization, family planning, and public health education. The AIDS epidemic and the apparent failure of conventional research approaches to an unconventional problem in unconventional populations has demanded new methodologies and the use of nontraditional approaches to knowledge generation.

The use of ethnography is a step forward in addressing these issues, but it is one to be taken with caution. Ethnographic methods must be adapted to fit the demands and requirements of action and intervention settings. Ethnographic evaluators must find rapid ways of collecting and analyzing qualitative and quantitative data that are graphic, readily understood, and sufficiently clear in their direction that they can be rapidly acted on by program administrators and staff.

In order to provide "condensed case studies," ethnographers must know more, not less. They must know enough about the type of program and its context to make rapid entry, to move quickly, to make critical and appropriate decisions about data collection, and to provide regular feedback in multiple areas of the program without being perceived as intrusive or as so comprehensive as to provide no direction.

Finally, ethnographers will be asked to make judgments. The best ethnographers in AIDS intervention programs will be those who understand programmatic responsibility and have both the experience and the data on which to base suggestions for program directions. The ethnographic method can make a major contribution to the struggle against AIDS. It will make that contribution only if anthropologists continue to shape the methodology to program and policy demands in collaboration with other researchers and program staff committed to innovative approaches to the AIDS challenge.

References

AIDS Community Research Group. *Knowledge, Attitudes, and Behavior in Hartford's Neighborhoods.* Hartford, Conn.: Institute for Community Research and ACRG Consortium, 1988.

AIDS Community Research Group. *Knowledge, Attitudes, and Behavior in Hartford's Neighborhoods.* Hartford, Conn.: Institute for Community Research and ACRG Consortium, 1989.

Antoniskis, D., Sattler, F. R., and Leedom, J. M. "Importance of Assessing Risk Behavior for AIDS." *Risk Assessment,* 1988, *83* (5), 138-160.

Barger, K., and Reza, E. "The Farmworker Movement in the Midwest." In D. Stull and J. J. Schensul (eds.), *Collaborative Research and Social Change: Applied Anthropology in Action.* Boulder, Colo.: Westview Press, 1987.

Becker, M. H., and Joseph, J. G. "AIDS and Behavioral Change to Reduce Risk: A Review." *American Journal of Public Health,* 1988, *78* (4), 394-410.

Bernard, H. R. *Research Methods in Cultural Anthropology.* Beverly Hills, Calif.: Sage, 1988.

Center for New Schools. "Ethnographic Evaluation in Education." *Journal of Research and Development in Education,* 1976, *9* (4), 3-11.

DiClemente, R. J., Boyer, C. B., and Morales, E. S. "Minorities and AIDS: Knowledge, Attitudes, and Misconceptions Among Black and Latino Adolescents." *American Journal of Public Health,* 1988, *78* (1), 55-57.

Downing, M. "Lesbian AIDS Project: An Ethnographic and Seroprevalence Study of Out-of-Treatment IVDUs in San Francisco." Paper presented at the Society for Applied Anthropology Meetings, Tampa, Florida, 1988.

Estrada, A. L., DeBoor, M., Fernandez, M., and Dalgorn, R. *AIDS Knowledge, Attitudes, Beliefs, and Behaviors: Preliminary Data Report from the University of Arizona—ADHS Minority AIDS Survey.* Tucson: College of Rural Health Office, University of Arizona, 1988.

Feldblum, P. J., and Fortney, J. A. "Condoms, Spermicides, and the Transmission of Human Immunodeficiency Virus: A Review of the Literature." *American Journal of Public Health,* 1988, *78* (1), 52-53.

Feldman, D. A., and Johnson, T. M. (eds.). *The Social Dimensions of AIDS.* New York: Praeger, 1986.

Fetterman, D. *Ethnography in Educational Evaluation.* Beverly Hills, Calif.: Sage, 1984.

Fineberg, H. V. "Education to Prevent AIDS: Prospects and Obstacles." *Science,* 1988, *239,* 592-596.

Fischl, M. A. "Prevention of Transmission of AIDS During Sexual Intercourse." In V. T. Pevita, S. Hellman, and S. A. Rosenberg (eds.), *AIDS: Etiology, Diagnosis, Treatment, and Prevention.* 2nd ed. Philadelphia: Lippincott, 1988.

Flam, R., and Stein, Z. "Behavior, Infection, and Immune Response: An Epidemiological Approach." In D. A. Feldman and T. M. Johnson (eds.), *The Social Dimensions of AIDS.* New York: Praeger, 1986.

Hispanic Health Alliance. *AIDS Knowledge, Attitudes, and Sexual Practices Among Hispanics in Chicago: Preliminary Results of a 1988 Citywide Survey.* Chicago: Illinois Department of Public Health, 1988.

Hopkins, D. R. "Public Health Measures for Prevention and Control of AIDS." *Measures/Outcomes,* 1987, *102* (5), 463-467.

Institute for Community Research. Project COPE internal documentation. Hartford, Conn.: Project COPE, Institute for Community Research, 1989.

LeCompte, M., and Goetz, J. "Ethnographic Data Collection in Evaluation Research." In D. Fetterman (ed.), *Ethnography in Educational Evaluation.* Beverly Hills, Calif.: Sage, 1984.

Mason, J. O., Noble, G., Lindsey, B., Kolbe, L., Van Ness, P., Bowen, G. S., Drotman, D. P., and Rosenberg, M. "Current CDC Efforts to Prevent and Control Human Immunodeficiency Virus Infection and AIDS in the United States Through Information and Education." *National AIDS Information/Education Program,* 1988, *103* (3), 255-260.

Page, J. B. "What You Know and What You Shoot With: Parenteral Drug Use and Risk of HIV Infection." Paper presented at the Society for Applied Anthropology Meetings, Tampa, Florida, April 1988.

Pelto, P. J., and Pelto, G. H. *Anthropological Research.* 2nd ed. New York: Cambridge University Press, 1978.

Peterson, J. L., and Morin, G. "Issues in the Prevention of AIDS Among Black and Hispanic Men." *American Psychologist,* 1988, 43 (11), 871–877.

Richwald, G. A., Schneider-Monoz, M., and Valdez, R. B. "Are Condom Instructions in Spanish Readable? Implications for AIDS Prevention Activities for Hispanics." *Hispanic Journal of Behavioral Sciences,* 1989, 11 (1), 70–82.

Rossi, P. H., and Freeman, H. E. *Evaluation: A Systematic Approach.* (4th ed.) Newbury Park, Calif.: Sage, 1989.

Schensul, S. L., and Schensul, J. J. "Advocacy and Applied Anthropology." In G. Weber and G. McCall (eds.), *Social Scientists as Advocates: Views from the Applied Disciplines.* Beverly Hills, Calif.: Sage, 1978.

Scrimshaw, S.C.M., and Hurtado, E. *Rapid Assessment Procedures for Nutrition and Primary Health Care: Anthropological Approaches to Improving Program Effectiveness.* Tokyo: United Nations University, 1988.

Selwyn, P. A., Feiner, C., Cox, C., Lipshutz, C., and Cohen, R. "Knowledge About AIDS and High-Risk Behavior Among Intravenous Drug Users in New York City." *Gower Academic Journals,* October 8, 1987, pp. 247–254.

Sevilla-Casa, E. *Malaria and Anthropology: Towards a Treatment of Malaric Communities as Human Ecosystems.* Bogotá, Colombia: University of Bogotá, 1989.

Sterk, C. "If You Want to Know, Talk with Us!" Paper presented at the Society for Applied Anthropology Meetings, Tampa, Florida, April 1988.

Stull, D., Grell, L. S., and Weston, T. *Kikapoo Nation: The Ways of Our People.* Powhattan, Kan.: Kikapoo Tribal Press, 1985.

Suchman, E. *Evaluative Research: Principles and Practice in Public Service and Social Action Programs.* New York: Russell Sage Foundation, 1967.

Weller, S. C., and Romney, A. K. *Systematic Data Collection, Volume 10: Qualitative Research Methods.* Newbury Park, Calif.: Sage, 1988.

Werner, O., and Schoepfle, G. M. *Systematic Fieldwork: Ethnographic Analysis and Data Management.* Beverly Hills, Calif.: Sage, 1987a.

Werner, O., and Schoepfle, G. M. *Systematic Fieldwork: Foundations of Ethnography and Interviewing.* Beverly Hills, Calif.: Sage, 1987b.

Wolcott, H. "Ethnographers Sans Ethnography: The Evaluation Compromise." In D. Fetterman (ed.), *Ethnography in Educational Evaluation.* Beverly Hills, Calif.: Sage, 1984.

Jean J. Schensul is a medical anthropologist, executive director of the Institute for Community Research, associate professor of anthropology at the University of Connecticut, and coprincipal investigator of Project COPE.

Stephen L. Schensul is a medical anthropologist, associate professor of community medicine, and director of the Center for International Community Health Studies at the University of Connecticut Medical School.

Lessons for AIDS preventive education can be drawn from research on public health problems of longer standing, such as smoking and drug abuse.

A Model for AIDS Education

Douglas Longshore

In response to a request from the Senate Governmental Affairs Committee, the U.S. General Accounting Office recently devised a model for preventive AIDS education and evaluated its applicability through field investigations of twelve "exemplary" AIDS prevention campaigns. The GAO's task was to identify the elements of effective AIDS education targeted specifically to three groups: intravenous drug users and their sex partners because of high rates of seroprevalence (Hahn, Onorato, Jones, and Dougherty, 1989); black and Latino populations because of the disproportionate number of cases from these groups (Curran, Jaffe, and Hardy, 1988); and adolescents because rates of infection are relatively high among those who are sexually active (Hein, 1988). Much of the existing evidence on AIDS education has measured the effectiveness of campaigns targeted to gay men (Office of Technology Assessment, 1988). Relatively little is known about the elements of effective AIDS education for other populations. Of course, there is a considerable body of research on public health problems of longer standing, such as smoking, drug use, and teenage pregnancy. The GAO drew on that research as well, and while the applicability of specific findings on other public health problems to AIDS prevention may be arguable, the GAO believed previous research could be instructive if implications were drawn with caution.

This chapter reviews the GAO model for AIDS education and compares it with models used in the development of other public health campaigns. The chapter synthesizes the lessons learned from these efforts into a sevenfactor model, which is illustrated with descriptions of twelve AIDS preven-

---

The views and opinions expressed by the author in this chapter are his own and should not be construed as the policy or position of the GAO.

tion campaigns identified by the GAO as "exemplary." Reflecting the Senate committee's interests, these campaigns are targeted to intravenous drug users, minorities, or youth. The model makes explicit the importance of providing actual risk-reduction skills and motivators. These factors are critical to prevention but have not been adequately emphasized in many AIDS prevention models now available.

Perhaps because of political constraints, guidance issued by the Centers for Disease Control (CDC) does not systematically identify the range of characteristics that can render a population at risk and offers little discussion of risk-reduction skills or motivators (Centers for Disease Control, 1987, 1988). While guidance from the social science community does cite all seven factors (allowing for variation in terminology and level of detail), underlying conceptual frameworks have not been made explicit, so the presumed importance of each factor and scope of the guidance often remain unclear (Coates, Stall, and Hoff, 1987; Fineberg, 1988; Joseph, 1987; McKusick, Conant, and Coates, 1985).

The work presented in this chapter relates to evaluation of AIDS prevention campaigns in several ways. First, it presents a consensus model on necessary program elements and desired outcomes. Second, until better evaluations of effectiveness are available, it presents a standard for comparison. Third, the GAO's effort to develop case studies of model efforts can be considered an initial evaluation of the state of development for campaigns directed at the target groups.

Identifying Model Campaigns

During the spring of 1988, the GAO staff conducted interviews with nationally recognized experts (academic researchers, practitioners, and policy advocates) in public health, community organization, mass communication, and marketing, as well as AIDS prevention and control. These experts were asked, first, to specify the elements they considered essential to effective public health interventions or marketing campaigns among the three populations specified by the Senate committee. Experts' responses, in combination with the GAO's review of relevant research literature, guided development of the seven-factor model.

Each expert then was asked to identify AIDS prevention campaigns that currently operated in any of the three U.S. cities hardest hit by AIDS— namely, Los Angeles, New York City, and San Francisco; that targeted drug users, minority communities, or adolescents; and that contained all the elements considered by the expert to be essential to effectiveness. Nominations converged on a set of twelve "exemplary" campaigns meant to reach one or more of the GAO's target groups (see Table 1).

During site visits, the GAO staff reviewed each campaign's rationale and operation, focusing on the design of AIDS prevention messages. In

Table 1. Model Campaigns and Target Groups

Campaign and City	Minority Groups	Intravenous Drug Users	Youth
AIDS Foundation, San Francisco	X	X	X
Association for Drug Abuse Prevention and Treatment, New York		X	
Bayview–Hunter's Point Foundation, San Francisco	X	X	
East Los Angeles Rape Hotline, Los Angeles	X		X
El Centro Human Services Corporation, Los Angeles	X	X	X
Health Watch, New York	X		X
Latino AIDS Project, San Francisco	X	X	X
MidCity Consortium to Combat AIDS, San Francisco		X	X
Minority AIDS Project, Los Angeles	X	X	X
Project Return, New York	X		
Stepping Stone, Los Angeles			X
The Wedge, San Francisco			X

most cases, data by which to evaluate campaign outcomes had not yet been systematically collected and analyzed, and the GAO's study was not designed to gather such data independently. Hence, the terms *exemplary* and *model* describe a campaign that, in the opinion of experts consulted by the GAO, is well designed and likely to be effective.

A Model for AIDS Education

When designing an AIDS prevention message, at least seven factors should be considered: (1) target group boundaries, (2) characteristics placing the group at risk, (3) media most likely to reach the group, (4) factual information appropriate to the group, (5) skills for risk reduction, (6) motivators for risk reduction, and (7) intended outcomes. It is important to note that this model pertains only to *message* design. It does not cover broader issues of *program* design, such as the value of conducting a baseline needs assessment, client involvement in decision making, or methods for evaluation and program revision.

Target Group. Is the plan to disseminate a broad message to all adolescents in the United States or a more particular message to inner-city youth or runaway teenagers who are homosexual; to reach all minority adults in New York City or mainly those at high risk for drug use? Previous public health experience suggests that the more precisely the target group is bounded, the more effective the campaign. Precision makes it easier to deliver a message that tells people exactly what they need to know, in their own language, through sources they trust and respect.

Community-based organizations have developed AIDS print media and seminars matched specifically to local populations. As an example, Health Watch runs an AIDS campaign targeted to Bedford-Stuyvesant adolescents and their parents. Local parents and youth have been closely involved in determining the content and style of two AIDS prevention brochures, one meant for parents and the other for teenagers. Focus-group discussions indicated that teens were not likely to accept sexual abstinence as a preventive measure unless the call for abstinence avoided moralism and emphasized teenagers' rights to make their own choices regarding sex. Both brochures reflected this advice.

Risk Characteristics. One reason for mounting a special AIDS education effort for some groups is the high incidence of risk behavior. Another aspect of the problem is that certain characteristics make it easier or more difficult for people to understand a health education message, characteristics such as educational background or familiarity with English. To address this issue, several of the GAO's model campaigns have developed brochures, comic books, and Spanish picture books called *novelas* that provide simple information on modes of transmission and ways to reduce risk. The material purposely is not so dense as to put off low-skill readers. A similar strategy is to put the bare essentials in headings or captions, so people unlikely to read every word can nonetheless get the gist of the message.

Research also indicates a need to consider characteristics associated with a group's sociopolitical attitudes and health practices. Few adolescents are well informed on techniques for contraception (Hein, 1988), and some immigrants to this country and users of illegal drugs actively avoid information sources connected with the government (Friedman, Des Jarlais, and Sotheran, 1987; Williams, 1986). In some minority communities, the AIDS threat is still met with considerable misunderstanding or denial. Even among homosexually active men, a message targeted expressly to "gay men" may not be effective if they do not use the term "gay" to describe themselves or if racial or ethnic identity is more salient to them than sexual preference (Williams, 1986).

Media. According to some research, blacks and Hispanics use television as an information source more than other groups, and radio is especially effective for reaching teenagers (Atkin, 1981; McGuire, 1985). On the other hand, regardless of the target group, mass media alone may be less effective in promoting behavior change than face-to-face contact or some combination of mass and personal media (Roberts and Maccoby, 1985). One means of face-to-face communication is the AIDS "social" or "house party" where an invitation-only meeting is held in a private home, during which professional health educators offers AIDS facts and safer-sex guidelines. Another face-to-face medium is the peer who speaks in the target group's own idiom, knows the local history, and is able to modulate the message, depending on a client's needs and reactions.

In some model campaigns, notably a school-based campaign called the Wedge, outreach staff include people who have AIDS. For obvious reasons, people with AIDS can be a credible source regarding the consequences of infection. And especially with school-based audiences, they may evoke compassion and cut through young people's presumption of invulnerability.

Factual Information. When education is targeted to well-defined groups, the message can be tailored accordingly. For intravenous drug users, it is important to describe fully the drug-related modes of virus transmission and, when users are interested in treatment, to describe the available treatment options. For young children, on the other hand, it might be enough to identify myths about transmission so that unfounded fears are dispelled. Older children can benefit from a lesson on various types of illness and the effects of AIDS on the human body, but the same lesson might leave intravenous drug users unimpressed.

Whatever facts are appropriate, they must be presented in a way that is readily understandable. As one expert put it, educating young people on AIDS without clearly discussing sex is like "trying to teach kids about baseball without mentioning the ball and glove" (U.S. General Accounting Office, 1988, p. 25). Yet the problem is not confined merely to young people. The GAO found considerable evidence that adults, too, have misunderstood clinical terms and euphemisms like "bodily fluids," misinterpreting "bodily fluids" to mean sweat and saliva (U.S. General Accounting Office, 1988).

To break through the misconception that AIDS is a disease that only infects white gay men, campaigns targeted to minority communities invoke symbols of family. Heterosexual families of color often appear in print materials. Even when the target group is minority drug users or minority homosexuals and bisexuals, the context is familial. In a skit offered by one Hispanic community theater group in Los Angeles, the scripted conversation among teens observes that "we're talking about protecting your sister, brother, your family."

Humor has also been used to convey factual information. Although it has not been shown to contribute directly to attitude change (McGuire, 1985), humor can lessen the discomfort associated with sensitive subjects, such as sexuality and death. A San Francisco AIDS Foundation bus poster reads in part, "You won't get AIDS from this bus or from bathrooms, giving blood, shaking hands, parakeets, old sneakers, microwaves, or spring cleaning." Other print media distributed by the San Francisco AIDS Foundation include a brochure with dancing condoms and "The Works," a comic book featuring cartoon viruses that speak.

Skills. Critical to effective AIDs education are actual skills that can be used to change behavior. Such skills, in part, are practical, including how and when a condom should be put on and taken off and how and when a drug user's works should be cleaned. Some model campaigns hand out illustrations of proper cleaning methods. Others actually demonstrate these methods for users who otherwise might not understand them.

Another set of critical skills is interpersonal—how to resist effectively the pressure to have sex, especially unprotected sex, or to use illegal drugs. Project Return in New York distributes a packet called "Use Condom Sense," with condom-wearing instructions, a sample condom, and a section on "how to talk to your partner." This section contains ten arguments against condoms and ten constructive answers. Outreach workers sit with a client, in the park, for instance, and together they practice these arguments and answers to help the client become more self-assured and more familiar with the concepts. Workers also stress the importance of agreeing on condom use or other safer-sex practices *before* sex is initiated.

Interpersonal skills can be nonverbal as well as verbal, and for some populations, such as low-income women, nonverbal skills may be more useful (Mays and Cochran, 1988). On the other hand, significant reductions in risk behavior have been reported among gay men who received training in verbal techniques of self-assertion (Kelly, St. Lawrence, and Hood, 1988).

Motivators. The degenerative and fatal nature of AIDs might seem to be sufficient motivation for behavior changes that reduce risk. But previous public health experience indicates that behavior is not greatly affected by low-probability events that occur only in the long term. What is the best way, then, to motivate risk reduction? One strategy is to emphasize the more immediate consequences of AIDS. The Health Watch brochure for teens warns that "AIDS can really mess you up" and cites as consequences the short-term symptoms and "ugly" lesions that are likely to create serious problems in a teenager's social life.

However, whether long-term or short-term consequences are cited, the motivating effect of fear may be limited (McGuire, 1985; Schott, 1986; Sutton, 1982). New York campaigns to reach drug users deliberately do not cite the alarming local statistics on AIDS incidence, but focus instead on the skills by which risk can be reduced. For populations not so vulnerable, fear may not be counterproductive if immediately paired with facts on risk reduction (McKusick, Conant, and Coates, 1985). In the educational skit offered by a Los Angeles campaign, one character observes that "this illness eats up your insides and then you're gonna dry up slowly. . . . Before you die, [AIDS] makes sure you remember *you had a choice*" (emphasis in original).

Prior research suggests several alternative positive motivators. One is normative support. For example, outreach campaigns for drug users attempt to set up a personal bond between worker and client so that over time a client becomes more reluctant to engage in risky behavior that would anger or disappoint the worker. Another normative motivator is a public commitment to risk reduction similar to that employed in public health interventions to reduce smoking and drug use (Polich, Ellickson, Reuter, and Kahan, 1984).

Self-reinforcement has also been utilized through a series of weekly group sessions. Kelly, St. Lawrence, and Hood (1988) trained gay men to generate and practice self-reinforcing statements such as "I will feel much better tomorrow if I don't do anything risky tonight" and "I am proud that I didn't do anything high in risk this week." The sessions also covered information on AIDS transmission, assertiveness training, and the encouragement of normative support from other group members. A comparison of experimental and control (waiting-list) subjects revealed significant risk behavior reductions among those trained.

"Eroticizing" is an effort to make safer-sex practices seem more attractive so that people can more easily substitute those practices for unprotected sex. The Bayview-Hunter's Point Foundation in San Francisco offers safer-sex kits including not one but three types of condoms, so people can easily experiment. This campaign also conducts seminars in which the adult audience is encouraged to become more comfortable with condoms by removing them from the package for close handling. Finally, exposure to video representations of safer sex, along with materials provided in person and print, have reportedly been more effective in promoting risk reduction among gay men than the oral and print materials alone (Quadland and others, n.d.).

Positive motivators can be more tangible as well, such as vouchers for getting into drug treatment programs and AIDS information brochures with a detachable questionnaire by which readers verify what they have learned. Readers submit the completed questionnaire as their entry in a sweepstakes. Drawn at random from those answering all items correctly, winners may be awarded prizes such as cash and condoms.

Intended Outcomes. For campaigns targeted to young children, the appropriate outcome may simply be more accurate knowledge of the modes of HIV transmission and nontransmission. Further information, such as details on risk behavior and risk-reduction methods, might only cause confusion and alarm (U.S. General Accounting Office, 1988). When targeting older children and adults, campaign designers may find it desirable to pursue multiple outcomes—both cognitive and behavioral. The domain of behavioral outcomes includes risk *prevention* among persons who still engage in illegal drug use or in unprotected sex and behavior *maintenance* among those whose habits have already changed.

In practice, however, message elements designed to achieve one outcome may undermine the effect of elements designed to achieve another (U.S. General Accounting Office, 1988). Some drug users, for example, may respond favorably to calls for the elimination of needle sharing, while others find that element of the message entirely unrealistic. If so, other elements describing proper procedures for needle cleaning may go unheeded.

Even when multiple outcomes are not discordant, it is still important to consider the precise needs of individuals within the target population. Messages designed to promote behavior change may be less than optimal for persons who have changed already. Such persons need information, skills, and motivators specifically designed to reduce the likelihood of relapse, an objective that appears much more difficult to achieve than initial change (Benfari, Ockene, and McIntyre, 1982). As another example, campaigns targeted to intravenous drug users are incomplete if they cover only the procedures necessary to prevent AIDS transmission during drug use. Though users now report cleaning their paraphernalia much more frequently, few say they have adopted safer-sex practices with their primary partners (Newmeyer, 1988). Thus, many who are HIV positive and who have eliminated the AIDS risk associated with drug use may still be transmitting the virus.

Comparison of AIDS with Other Public Health Issues

AIDS education shares several common elements with previous public health campaigns. First, it is clear that campaigns using mass media alone can raise issue salience and provide basic information to a wide public audience. Second, however, it is also clear that sustained, intense contact is necessary to influence actual behavior. Such contact can be mediated in part. The GAO's model campaigns used skits and videos to spark personal discussion afterward, but messages sent through mass media alone will probably not be enough to get people at risk to take steps that will lower their risk.

Third, factual information about how to reduce AIDS risk should cover outcome efficacy, defined as information about the effectiveness of those measures (McKusick, Conant, and Coates, 1985; Schott, 1986). People also need to practice a skill in advance so they will know they can carry it out. This mastery of the skill also offers a clear sense of personal efficacy (McKusick, Conant, and Coates, 1985; Schott, 1986).

Fourth, the use of fear is problematic but not necessarily unwise. It can raise dramatically the salience of an issue, rendering audience members more eager to know how to reduce their risk. Fear may also be helpful in producing behavior change if a moderate but not high level of fear is aroused, if the message focuses on short-term consequences or personalizes long-term consequences, and if the message also cites specific ways to reduce risk (Sutton, 1982).

On the other hand, AIDS education has several elements that distinguish it from other public health campaigns. First, AIDS risk behaviors are stigmatized, and many members of high-risk groups are underground. Therefore, it is essential to route AIDS education through indigenous sources, including informal street communication networks and peer cadres, such as former drug users. It is also important to focus on risk behaviors, not risk categories, since many people at risk are not in those categories, and many who are do not see themselves in those terms.

Second, many people at risk for AIDS are not accustomed to handling conflict through mutual self-disclosure. For them, it may be important to develop nonverbal as well as verbal skills; for example, they may need guidance in creating and exploiting just the right moment to put on a condom. Third, because many at-risk people have low reading skills, educational materials must be designed to convey information in pictures and simple words. For example, the CDC's 1988 national mail-out brochure was reportedly written at an eighth-grade level, well above the skills of many readers of English, let alone readers for whom English is not their primary language.

Conclusion

AIDS prevention messages appropriate to groups at higher risk should cover at least seven factors: target group boundaries, characteristics placing the group at risk, media likely to reach the group, factual information appropriate to the group, skills for risk reduction, motivators for risk reduction, and intended outcomes. Evaluations of such messages should be based on this or a similar model. The first six factors should be made operational as measures of mediating (or intermediate outcome) variables. Intended outcomes should be tailored to the target groups and the dynamics of behavior change.

References

Atkin, C. K. "Mass Media Information Campaign Effectiveness." In R. E. Rice and W. J. Pailsey (eds.), *Public Communication Campaigns*. Beverly Hills, Calif.: Sage, 1981.

Benfari, R. C., Ockene, J. K., and McIntyre, K. M. "Control of Cigarette Smoking from a Psychological Perspective." *Annual Review of Public Health*, 1982, 3, 101-128.

Centers for Disease Control. *Guidelines for AIDS Prevention Program Operations.* Atlanta, Ga.: U.S. Department of Health and Human Services, 1987.
Centers for Disease Control. "Guidelines for Effective School Health Education to Prevent the Spread of AIDS." *Morbidity and Mortality Weekly Report,* 1988, *37* (S-2), 1-14.
Coates, T. J., Stall, R. D., and Hoff, C. C. *Changes in Sexual Behavior Among Gay and Bisexual Men Since the Beginning of the AIDS Epidemic.* Washington, D.C.: Office of Technology Assessment, 1987.
Curran, J. W., Jaffe, H. W., and Hardy, A. M. "Epidemiology of the HIV Infection and AIDS in the United States." *Science,* 1988, *239,* 610-616.
Fineberg, H. V. "Education to Prevent AIDS: Prospects and Obstacles." *Science,* 1988, *239,* 592-596.
Friedman, S. R., Des Jarlais, D. C., and Sotheran, J. L. "AIDS and Self-Organization Among Intravenous Drug Users." *International Journal of the Addictions,* 1987, *22* (3), 201-219.
Hahn, R. A., Onorato, I. M., Jones, T. S., and Dougherty, J. "Prevalence of HIV Infection Among Intravenous Drug Users in the United States." *Journal of the American Medical Association,* 1989, *261* (18), 2677-2684.
Hein, K. "AIDS in Adolescents: Exploring the Challenge." Unpublished paper, Columbia University, 1988.
Joseph, J. *HIV Infection and the Effectiveness of Education for the "General Population."* Washington, D.C.: Office of Technology Assessment, 1987.
Kelly, J. A., St. Lawrence, J., and Hood, J. S. "Behavioral Intervention to Reduce AIDS Risk Activities." Paper presented at the Fourth Annual International Conference on AIDS, Stockholm, Sweden, June 12-16, 1988.
McGuire, W. J. "Attitudes and Attitude Change." In G. Lindzey and E. Aronson (eds.), *Handbook of Social Psychology.* Vol. 2. 3rd ed. New York: Random House, 1985.
McKusick, L., Conant, M., and Coates, T. J. "The AIDS Epidemic: A Model for Developing Intervention Strategies for Reducing High-Risk Behavior in Gay Men." *Sexually Transmitted Diseases,* 1985, *12* (4), 229-234.
Mays, V. M., and Cochran, S. D. "Issues in the Perception of AIDS Risk and Risk Reduction Activities by Black and Hispanic/Latina Women." *American Psychologist,* 1988, *43* (11), 949-957.
Newmeyer, J. "Why Bleach? Fighting AIDS Contagion Among IV Drug Users: The San Francisco Experience." In R. J. Battjes and R. W. Pickens (eds.), *Needle Sharing Among Intravenous Drug Users: National and International Perspectives.* NIDA Research Monograph, no. 80. Washington, D.C.: U.S. Government Printing Office, 1988.
Office of Technology Assessment. *How Effective Is AIDS Education?* Washington, D.C.: Office of Technology Assessment, 1988.
Polich, J. M., Ellickson, P. L., Reuter, P., and Kahan, J. P. *Strategies for Controlling Adolescent Drug Use.* Santa Monica, Calif.: Rand, 1984.
Quadland, M. C., Shattls, W., Schuman, R., Jacobs, R., and D'Eramo, J. *The 800 Men Study: A Systematic Evaluation of AIDS Prevention Programs.* New York: The 800 Men Project Staff, 1987.
Roberts, D. F., and Maccoby, N. "Effects of Mass Communication." In G. Lindzey and E. Aronson (eds.), *Handbook of Social Psychology.* Vol. 2. 3rd ed. New York: Random House, 1985.
Schott, J. R. "Psychosocial Reactions to Acquired Immune Deficiency Syndrome (AIDS) in Two Populations at Risk." Unpublished doctoral dissertation, California School of Professional Psychology, 1986.

Sutton, S. R. "Fear-Arousing Communications: A Critical Examination of Theory and Research." In J. R. Eiser (ed.), *Social Psychology and Behavioral Medicine*. New York: Wiley, 1982.

U.S. General Accounting Office. *AIDS Education: Reaching Populations at Higher Risk*. Program Evaluation and Methodology Division, no. 88-35. Washington, D.C.: U.S. General Accounting Office, 1988.

Williams, L. S. "AIDS Risk Reduction: A Community Health Education Intervention for Minority High-Risk Group Members." *Health Education Quarterly*, 1986, *13* (4), 407-421.

Douglas Longshore was a project manager with the U.S. General Accounting Office from 1984 to 1989 and is now project director with the Drug Abuse Research Group at the Neuropsychiatric Institute, University of California, Los Angeles.

Three theoretical approaches to disease prevention and health promotion are discussed and an example of an AIDS prevention curriculum that used theories to formulate the intervention and to guide the evaluation research is presented.

Theory-Based Evaluation of AIDS-Related Knowledge, Attitudes, and Behavior Changes

Ross F. Conner, Shiraz I. Mishra, Megan A. Lewis, Samantha Bryer, Jeff Marks, Mini Lai, Lisa Clark

The AIDS crisis has challenged researchers in a variety of professions to develop effective measures to assist those already infected with the HIV virus and to stop the spread of the virus to susceptible but currently uninfected individuals. In the case of those who are HIV positive or who have clinical AIDS, biomedical research has developed techniques to identify the virus and ameliorative protocols (Schwartz, Dans, and Kinosian, 1988; Surbone and others, 1988; Wainberg, Kendall, and Gilmore, 1988). With this same group, social science research is helping to identify factors that facilitate the psychological adjustment of those individuals with AIDS, as well as those associated or working with people with AIDS (Coates and others, 1987; Hull, 1987; Klein, 1988).

In the case of the large population of individuals who are susceptible to the virus but currently HIV negative, the only preventive measure available for the foreseeable future is a social-psychological one. People must be educated to change their AIDS-related knowledge, attitudes, and behaviors (Becker and Joseph, 1988; Fineberg, 1988; Valdiserri and others, 1987). Professionals who are developing and evaluating these AIDS prevention

---

This chapter was first presented at the American Evaluation Association annual meeting in October 1988. We gratefully acknowledge those who have assisted us in various ways during this project: Dr. Hung Fan, Dr. Luis Villareal, Jefferie Jimerez, and Michelle Richards.

programs can draw on a tradition of theory in the disease prevention and health promotion areas. This chapter discusses these theories and presents an example of an AIDs prevention program that used the theories to formulate the intervention and to guide the evaluation research.

The Theoretical Bases

Attempts to understand why people do or do not engage in a variety of health-related behaviors has a fairly long history. Over the years, the theories and models aimed at understanding these behaviors have become increasingly complex and sophisticated (Wallston and Wallston, 1984). Consequently, there are a variety of theories and models from a number of disciplines that provide insights to guide the development and evaluation of disease prevention programs, whether they focus on AIDS, diet changes, or smoking behavior (Fishbein and Ajzen, 1975; Farquhar, 1978).

Health Belief Model. The Health Belief Model (HBM) was formulated to understand the widespread failure of people to accept disease prevention techniques or screening tests for early detection of asymptomatic diseases (Rosenstock, 1966, 1974). The components of this theory were derived from an established body of literature that indicated that behavior depended primarily on two factors: the personal value placed on a particular goal and a person's estimate of the likelihood that a certain behavior could help achieve that goal (Becker, 1974; Becker and Maiman, 1983).

Translated into the context of health-related behavior, these factors indicate a person's desire to avoid illness or, if already ill, to get well and the belief that a specific health action will prevent or ameliorate an illness or disease. Specifically, the HBM consists of three main dimensions: perceived susceptibility, perceived severity, and the evaluation of an advocated or recommended behavior. The HBM has served as a major organizing framework for explaining and predicting acceptance of health and medical recommendations and has received support in both retrospective and prospective studies examining preventive health behaviors (Janz and Becker, 1984).

Health Decision Model. The Health Decision Model (HDM) is a recent reformulation of the HBM that attempts to approximate more closely the actual context in which decisions are made regarding health-related behavioral changes (Eraker, Becker, Strecher, and Kirscht, 1985). This model incorporates the three dimensions of perceived severity, susceptibility, and evaluation of a recommended behavior and also highlights the importance of experience, knowledge, and social interaction, among other areas. By adding these dimensions to the HBM formulation, theorists came closer to approximating the process of a person deciding to change behaviors that increase the risk for illness and disease.

Neither of these two models attempts to address the dynamic nature of the process of actual behavioral change. Both the HBM and the HDM are static in their formulation of health behavior change. The process of behavioral change is especially important regarding AIDS-related behaviors since the decision to engage in safe-sex practices involves important emotional, psychological, and social consequences. For example, the decision to use condoms may engender fears or the realization that one may be at risk for a dreadful and deadly disease.

Precaution-Adoption Process Model. The Precaution-Adoption Process Model (PAP) highlights the process of deciding to change health-related behaviors and recognizes the dynamic nature of these changes (Weinstein, 1988). The PAP model is unique in that it views behavior change as a dynamic process and is sensitive to the shifting nature in which decisions to make behavioral changes take place. The model proposes that people go through five stages in the behavior-change process. The first stage is mere knowledge about the risk. The second stage is characterized by the belief that there is a significant risk for other people, while the third stage is an acknowledgment of some personal susceptibility. The fourth stage represents the decision to take a precaution to reduce risk, and the fifth involves the actual steps taken to reduce risk. Each of the stages has specific determinants associated with it (such as knowledge about the seriousness of the risk or experience with the risk) that build on previous determinants as a person progresses through the stages. Thus, each stage is a cumulative experience of those preceding, but movement through the stages can be forward or backward as a person's knowledge, intentions, emotions, values, and actions change over time.

Application of Theory to an AIDS Prevention Program

We incorporated aspects of the HBM, the HDM, and the PAP model to develop an intervention and an associated evaluation. Thus, important theoretical concepts from the three models, such as knowledge, personal vulnerability, perceived susceptibility, role of social interaction, and the dynamic nature of the behavioral change process, were incorporated into the intervention program and guided the selection of the evaluation measures.

The intervention was a ten-week AIDS education class entitled "AIDS Fundamentals," offered during spring 1988 at the University of California, Irvine. The AIDS Fundamentals class was taught from a multidisciplinary perspective through the Social Ecology Program and the Molecular Biology and Biochemistry Department. The class covered topics related to the biological, epidemiological, psychosocial, legal, and ethical aspects of the AIDS epidemic, as well as practical information related to disease transmission, condom use, and safer sexual practices. Furthermore, two class sessions were devoted to individuals dealing directly with the AIDS crisis. People with AIDS formed one guest panel, and individuals working with people with AIDS comprised the second panel. Finally, the class involved personal, peer-led, small-group discussion sessions. The small-group discussion sessions served as a forum to address the students' fears, attitudes, and misconceptions in a nonthreatening environment.

Procedure. We used a one-group pretest-posttest design for this intervention. The pretest survey was given to the students on the first day of class, and the posttest survey was given at the end of the last class, ten weeks later. To ensure confidentiality, we had students create their own unique secret code to help match their pre- and posttest surveys.

Sample. Participants for this evaluation were drawn from 154 students enrolled for the spring 1988 offering of the class. From this group, seventy-five students voluntarily participated in the pretest and 101 students in the posttest. Pretest participation was lower than the posttest presumably because the survey, besides being optional, contained sensitive and personal questions. In addition, it was long and was handed out on the first day of class; thus, the students may not have realized that there might be personal benefits from their participation. The higher response rate at the posttest could be attributed to a higher awareness and an increased sense of the seriousness of the topics under discussion. Furthermore, by the end of the course, most of the sensitive topics had been discussed openly in class or in the informal small-group discussion sessions. The results presented in this section will focus on the sample of fifty-one students who participated at the pre- and posttest assessments of the evaluation.

Our sample represents 33 percent of the class. Based on demographic characteristics from the whole class, the sample is comparable to the entire class on age, ethnicity, and marital status. There were small differences in gender distribution, class level, and sexual experience (see Table 1).

Measures. Students completed a nine-page, 149-item questionnaire that contained questions assessing their AIDS-related knowledge, opinions and attitudes, behaviors, personal and interpersonal experiences, and demographic characteristics. The items on knowledge, opinions, and attitudes were adapted from Rhodes and Wolitski (n.d.).

AIDS-related knowledge was assessed by thirty-five questions that covered the domains of modes of transmission, epidemiology, preventive measures, severity of disease, and pathological extent of the disease. These questions were scored using a five-point scale incorporating the respondents' judgments of true versus false and the certainty of their judgment.

The five domains of AIDS-related opinions and attitudes were measured using thirty-four questions. These five domains assessed students' perceptions of such issues as desire for information, personal susceptibility, importance of social norms, severity of disease, and the effectiveness of preventive interventions. These questions were rated using a seven-point scale with responses ranging from strong agreement to strong disagreement.

AIDS-related behaviors and intentions for changing these behaviors

Table 1. Demographic Characteristics of the AIDS Fundamentals Class and the Study Sample

Characteristics	Class[a] (n = 128)	Sample (n = 51)
	Mean Years	
Age	22.1	21.9
Ethnicity	Percentages	
Anglo	52.8	58.8
Asian	31.2	29.4
Latino	9.6	7.8
Black	4.0	2.0
Other	2.4	2.0
Marital Status		
Never married	90.5	94.1
Married	6.3	5.9
Divorced, separated, widowed	3.2	0.0
Gender		
Female	62.5	76.5
Male	37.5	23.5
Class Level		
Senior	50.0	52.9
Junior	22.7	15.7
Sophomore	15.6	21.6
Freshman	8.6	7.8
Previous Sexual Experience		
Yes	71.4	62.0
No	28.6	38.0

[a] There were 128 students out of a total of 154 who voluntarily completed the demographic survey.

were measured by fifty-one questions. These questions inquired into the students' sexual activities, drug use habits, and AIDS-related personal experiences with friends or significant others. Most of these questions used a yes or no response category. The remaining questions inquired into the students' perceptions of susceptibility of various groups of people based on either their ethnicity, age, or sexual orientation and about their demographic characteristics.

Results. This section presents pre- and posttest scores on the measures that assessed the important theoretical dimensions guiding the intervention and evaluation. These dimensions include desire for information, perception of the severity of disease threat, perceived availability and ease of implementation of ameliorative strategies, opinions of others concerning these strategies, and perceived effectiveness of these strategies. In addition, the sample is characterized according to the PAP model stages.

AIDS-Related Knowledge. Using the most conservative assessment of knowledge gain, we noted a significant change of thirty-two points in the knowledge score between the two assessments (see Table 2). From a pretest low of 94, the knowledge score improved to 126 at the posttest, with a 50 percent decrease in the posttest standard deviation. This improvement in the absolute knowledge scale score reflects a gain of positive facts about the AIDS epidemic.

AIDS-Related Opinions and Attitudes. As the following list shows, some attitudes and opinions changed, while others did not.

1. Desire for information: At the pretest, the sample as a whole had a strong desire for AIDS-related information, and this trend continued at the posttest. Furthermore, as seen in Table 2, the means of 6.4 and 6.2 at the two time points, respectively, were close to the strongest possible endorsement of the desire to acquire information pertaining to many aspects of the AIDS epidemic.

2. Personal susceptibility: There was a small but significant change on this variable from pre- to posttest, from a neutral position to a slight decrease in a sense of personal susceptibility.

3. Importance of social norms: At both pre- and posttests, students moderately agreed with the idea that there were clear social norms about desirable AIDS-related behaviors.

4. Effectiveness of preventive measures: At the pretest, students mildly agreed that current AIDS-related preventive measures were effective. There was a significant increase in the endorsement of the effectiveness of these preventive behaviors and practices at the posttest.

Table 2. Mean Scores on AIDS-Related Knowledge, Opinions, and Attitudes Scales[a]

	Means (s.d.)	
	Pretest	Posttest
Knowledge Scale		
Group score	93.9 (17.9)	125.5 (8.6)[b]
Actual range	41–129	105–138
Possible range	35–140	35–140
AIDS-Related Opinions and Attitudes: Domains[c]		
Desire for information	6.4 (0.6)	6.2 (0.7)
Personal susceptibility	4.0 (1.1)	3.6 (1.0)[b]
Perception of social norms	4.8 (0.9)	4.8 (0.9)
Preventive effectiveness	4.8 (1.1)	5.8 (0.9)[b]
Severity of disease	4.7 (1.1)	4.6 (1.3)

[a] $n = 51$
[b] $p < 0.05$
[c] Scores range from 1 to 7, with 1 indicating strong disagreement, 4 a neutral position, and 7 indicating strong agreement.

5. Severity of disease: The scores at the two time points indicated that the students only mildly agreed that the consequences of AIDs were extremely severe.

Precaution-Adoption Process Model Stages. We used scores on the major determinants of each of the five PAP stages to characterize the class in terms of knowledge about AIDS (stage 1), acknowledgment of the risk for others (stage 2) or self (stage 3), intention to change one's AIDS-related behaviors (stage 4), and achievement of these changes (stage 5).

The first stage of this model involves a recognition of the AIDS risk. As previously discussed, students had a fairly high level of knowledge about the risks and consequences of AIDS. This finding was especially evident at the posttest where the score was 126 out of a possible 140. Thus, the large majority of students were well into or beyond the first stage of the PAP model.

The second stage involves the acknowledgment of a high level of susceptibility to AIDS for other people. Table 3 shows the means and standard deviations on questions that were representative of the determinants of this stage, as well as for the subsequent stages. There was a high degree of agreement at the pre- and posttests that some people (injection drug users and gay men) were at a high level of susceptibility. Thus, many students in the sample acknowledged that some people have a high level of risk for AIDS, indicating that most students were well into or had progressed beyond stage two.

Table 3. Precaution-Adoption Process Model Stage Scores: Means and Correlations[a]

	Means (s.d.) Pretest	Means (s.d.) Posttest
Stage 2: Acknowledging High Risk for Others[b]		
People who use intravenous drugs are at high risk for AIDS	6.8 (0.4)	7.0 (0.1)
Gay men are at high risk for AIDS	6.8 (0.7)	6.7 (0.8)
Stage 3: Personal Susceptibility[b]		
I consider my own risk to be very low	5.5 (1.4)	5.7 (1.6)
I am not worried about getting AIDS	3.8 (2.0)	3.9 (1.8)

	Correlations Pretest	Correlations Posttest
Stage 4: Intentions to Change Behavior		
Personal susceptibility × Intentions to take action	–0.04	0.31
Stage 5: Action Taken		
Intentions to take action × Actions taken	0.16	0.42[c]

[a] $n = 51$

[b] Scores range from 1 to 7, with 1 indicating strong disagreement, 4 a neutral position, and 7 indicating strong agreement.

[c] $p < 0.05$

The next stage of this model is acknowledgment of personal susceptibility to AIDS. In general, the students perceived their own susceptibility to be moderately low. As seen in Table 3, on an average students considered their own AIDS risk to be low and were not worried about getting AIDS. Thus, few students were at this stage of the process.

The fourth stage focuses specifically on one's intentions to make behavioral changes once one has acknowledged personal susceptibility. Since a minority of students viewed themselves as susceptible, it is most instructive to analyze the relationship between degree of personal susceptibility and intention to take action. As seen in Table 3, there was effectively no relationship between these two dimensions at the pretest and a positive, stronger relationship ($r = 0.31$) after the course. These findings indicate that a small proportion of students had reached stage four of the model.

The final stage of this model involves converting intentions into actions and adopting preventive measures to safeguard against the risk of AIDS. To test this, we correlated intention to take action with self-reported actions taken. The correlation was positive but low at the pretest and positive and significantly stronger at the posttest. This finding indicated that some students, then, were at the final stage of the PAP model, attempting the difficult transition from good intentions to meaningful preventive behaviors.

Discussion. This evaluation documented changes in AIDS-related knowledge, attitudes, behavioral intentions, and behaviors that occurred over the course of a ten-week educational intervention with college students. Because we used a one-group design, we cannot state with certainty that these changes were caused by the intervention. The types and direction of changes, however, were uniformly consistent with the changes we sought and the changes we would predict from the theoretical models that underlay the intervention. In a follow-up study of the next offering of the course, we used a quasi-experimental design with a comparison group to evaluate more definitively the outcomes of the class. These analyses are now under way.

In drawing conclusions about the effects of the current intervention, therefore, we must recognize that our design precludes definitive cause-and-effect statements linking program components with measured changes. Nonetheless, we can identify several outcomes that can inform future research and that we are currently exploring with the data from our quasi-experimental evaluation.

At the end of the AIDS Fundamentals class, students had a higher level of knowledge regarding various facets of the AIDS epidemic. In addition, we believed their attitudes concerning the various issues related to AIDS were generally of a more productive nature. This change can be seen in the more realistic view of their own susceptibility, a high level of continued interest in facts about AIDS, and their acknowledgment of the existence of preventive measures that can be taken against the AIDS virus.

Furthermore, students seem well into the process of initiating action to change their behavior according to the PAP model. Most students had surpassed the first stage of the model (knowledge) and had progressed to acknowledging personal susceptibility for some other people, namely, injection drug users and gay men. Many students, however, did not acknowledge that their own susceptibility might be high. This perception is a realistic assessment based on the reported sexual orientation and sexual experience of most class members. In addition, there is evidence to suggest that by the end of the class, those students who felt greater personal susceptibility were also those who had stronger intentions to change their behavior. More important in terms of AIDS prevention, at the end of the course, those who had stronger intentions to change their behavior were also those more likely to report having taken preventive actions.

Assessing changes due specifically to the class was only one purpose of the current study. Another important purpose was to adapt the dimensions shown in past research to be important components in disease prevention and health promotion programs to the case of an AIDS education and prevention intervention. In addition, we wanted to explore the feasibility of tracking the process of behavior change according to a newly formulated health behavioral change model. In general, we were able to adapt these dimensions successfully and, at least at a group level, to track the behavior-change process.

The structure and nature of the course, however, hindered the ideal application and evaluation of the theoretical dimensions. For example, because of the dynamic nature of the process, the PAP model requires a repeated-measure design, with frequent measures over a long time period. We were only able to take two measurements, one at the outset of the intervention and another at its conclusion ten weeks later. We would have liked to have monitored each individual's change process during the ten weeks, as well as over the subsequent months. We attempted a follow-up approximately two months after the end of the intervention, but the low response rate made the data unusable.

Conclusion

Education is currently the only tool available in preventing the spread of AIDS. Because of the dire consequences that result from ineffective programs, it is especially important both to draw on previous theory and research in developing programs and to evaluate the programs once they are implemented. Theory-based evaluation can guide future program development and evaluation by identifying the dimensions that are most important in facilitating and inhibiting behavior change.

References

Becker, M. H. (ed.). "The Health Belief Model and Personal Health Behavior." *Health Education Monographs*, 1974, 2 (4), entire issue.

Becker, M. H., and Joseph, J. G. "AIDS and Behavioral Change to Reduce Risk: A Review." *American Journal of Public Health,* 1988, *78* (4), 394-410.
Becker, M. H., and Maiman, L. A. "Models of Health-Related Behavior." In D. Mechanic (ed.), *Handbook of Health, Health Care, and the Health Professions.* New York: Free Press, 1983.
Coates, T. J., Stall, R., Mandel, J. S., Boccellari, A., Sorensen, J. L., Morales, E. F., Morin, S. F., Wiley, J. A., and McKusick, L. "AIDS: A Psychosocial Research Agenda." *Annals of Behavioral Medicine,* 1987, *9* (2), 21-28.
Eraker, S. A., Becker, M. H., Strecher, V. J., and Kirscht, J. P. "Smoking Behavior Cessation Techniques and the Health Decision Model." *American Journal of Medicine,* 1985, *78,* 817-825.
Farquhar, J. W. "The Community-Based Model of Life-Style Intervention Trials." *American Journal of Epidemiology,* 1978, *108* (2), 103-111.
Fineberg, H. V. "Education to Prevent AIDS: Prospects and Obstacles." *Science,* 1988, *239,* 592-596.
Fishbein, M., and Ajzen, I. *Beliefs, Attitude, Intention, and Behavior: An Introduction to Theory and Research.* Reading, Mass.: Addison-Wesley, 1975.
Hull, F. "The Role of Sociobehavioral Scientists in Health Care Practice." *Social Science and Medicine,* 1987, *25* (6), 679-687.
Janz, N. K., and Becker, M. H. "The Health Belief Model: A Decade Later." *Health Education Quarterly,* 1984, *11,* 1-47.
Klein, R. "Low Occupational Risk of Human Immunodeficiency Virus Infection Among Dental Professionals." *New England Journal of Medicine,* 1988, *318* (2), 86-90.
Rhodes, F., and Wolitski, R. J. *Factor Analytically Based Surveys for Measuring AIDS Knowledge and Attitudes.* Preliminary project report. Long Beach: California State University, n.d.
Rosenstock, I. M. "Why People Use Health Services." *Milbank Memorial Fund Quarterly,* 1966, *44,* 94-124.
Rosenstock, I. M. "The Health Belief Model and Preventive Health Behavior." *Health Education Monographs,* 1974, *2,* 354-386.
Schwartz, J., Dans, P. E., and Kinosian, B. P. "Human Immunodeficiency Virus Test Evaluation, Performance, and Use." *Journal of the American Medical Association,* 1988, *259* (17), 2574-2579.
Surbone, A., Yarchoan, R., McAtee, N., Blum, M. R., Maha, M., Allain, J-P., Thomas, R. V., Mitsuya, H., Lehrman, S. N., Leuther, M., Pluda, J. M., Jacobsen, F. K., Kessler, H. A., Myers, C. E., and Broder, S. "Treatment of the Acquired Immune Deficiency Syndrome (AIDS) and AIDS-Related Complex with a Regimen of 3'-azido-2', 3'-Dideoxythymidine (Azidothymidine or Zidovudine), and Acyclovir: A Pilot Study." *Annals of Internal Medicine,* 1988, *108* (4), 534-540.
Valdiserri, R. O., Lyter, D. W., Leviton, L. C., Stoner, K., and Silvestre, A. "Applying the Criteria for the Development of Health Promotion and Education Programs to AIDS Risk-Reduction Programs for Gay Men." *Journal of Community Health,* 1987, *12* (4), 199-212.
Wainberg, M. A., Kendall, O., and Gilmore, N. "Vaccine and Antiviral Strategies Against Infections Caused by Human Immunodeficiency Virus." *Canadian Medical Association Journal,* 1988, *138* (9), 797-807.
Wallston, B. S., and Wallston, K. A. "Social Psychological Models of Health Behavior: An Examination and Integration." In A. Baum, S. E. Taylor, and J. E. Singer (eds.), *Handbook of Psychology and Health.* Vol. 4. Hillsdale, N.J.: Erlbaum, 1984.
Weinstein, N. D. "The Precaution-Adoption Process." *Health Psychology,* 1988, *7* (4), 355-386.

Ross F. Conner is president of the American Evaluation Association and associate professor in the Social Ecology Program and the Public Policy Research Organization at the University of California, Irvine.

Shiraz I. Mishra is a doctoral student in the Social Ecology Program at the University of California, Irvine.

Megan A. Lewis is a doctoral student in the Social Ecology Program at the University of California, Irvine.

Samantha Bryer, Jeff Marks, Mini Lai, and Lisa Clark are undergraduate students at the University of California, Irvine, who participated in the AIDS Fundamentals class and in the research program.

This chapter presents strategies for developing, implementing, and evaluating effective AIDS prevention programs within the confines of a partnership between an evaluator and a target community.

AIDS Prevention Programs: The Need for Evaluation in the Context of Community Partnership

Joanne E. Mantell, Anthony T. DiVittis

In the absence of early governmental public health interventions in the United States, AIDS prevention strategies initially were implemented by community-based organizations (CBOs) and were targeted largely at white middle-class men who have sex with men. This early response has broadened, however, and a panoply of AIDS education and prevention programs now exist for other groups with high-risk behaviors, groups that exist within other social networks. Historically, AIDS health promotion has been heavily oriented toward individual behavioral change, while attempts to change sources of social influence or group and community social norms have been minimal. Therefore, the long-term maintenance of behavioral changes is in question.

AIDS prevention programs have taken a course similar to that of other social programs in that few are evaluated initially with scientific rigor. Evaluation activities have been limited for a number of reasons, including competition with direct clinical and educational services for funding, perceived lack of importance, lack of staff resources, and antiresearch sentiments. In addition, because of the urgency of the need, prevention programs have often been designed hastily, based on trial and error rather than on planning driven by social and behavioral science theories. There is a perception that offering some program is better than having no program to offer. This crisis mentality has led to the absence of systematic evaluation planning for most AIDS prevention programs.

Some health professionals prefer intrusive infection-containment measures, such as an "HIV parole system" (Archer, 1989), quarantine under certain circumstances (Judson, 1989), and nonvoluntary partner notification (Potterat, Spencer, Woodhouse, and Muth, 1989), rather than more conservative preventive education programs. As there is limited evaluation of the costs and benefits of these two approaches, one can only conjecture which is more effective. Based on our experience, we believe that one of the most effective solutions to the problem of reducing HIV risk behaviors is the implementation of effective AIDS prevention programs. Effectiveness is best determined when evaluation strategies are incorporated into the program strategy. Community involvement is essential. A partnership between the evaluator and the target community provides a framework that can facilitate evaluation.

Working with Communities and Community-Based Organizations

Benefits of Collaborative Evaluation. Communities under siege, faced with overwhelming problems other than AIDS and dire needs for direct services, often will not set a high priority for rigorous program evaluation because of their focus on competition for scarce resources. In addition, overcoming obstacles to the conduct of research will be difficult in poor, ethnic or racial minority, and medically disenfranchised communities that feel that research, policy, and resource agendas are not of their making. For example, involuntary sterilization experiments on incarcerated syphilis patients and the administration of hepatitis B vaccine to the institutionalized developmentally disabled have hurt the credibility of public health with these groups. Implementation of program evaluation may also be deterred by a political or cultural climate in which a moral judgment is attached to a public health problem (Freudenberg, Lee, and Silver, 1989). For example, denial of the existence of male-to-male anal intercourse among Hispanics may compel community leaders to object to including this variable in a program evaluation instrument.

Community mobilization and development may provide the means by which AIDS prevention programs and their assessment are promoted (Braithwaite and Lythcott, 1989). But before cooperating or committing resources, communities and their CBOs need to understand how research can benefit their constituency. People must be involved in identifying their needs and setting prevention priorities. Thus, a major task for the evaluator is to educate a community and any relevant agencies about the benefits of program evaluation.

Evaluation can benefit a community or CBO in several ways. First, it can be marketed as a tool for facilitating community empowerment. Through collective participation in program assessment, community members' sense of control over doing something to combat AIDS may be enhanced. Second, program evaluation and monitoring provide a means of accountability. Evaluation results can be used to alert funding sources to unmet needs or to convince them to fund additional phases of the evaluated program or new types of programs. Third, evaluation can provide a forum for program information feedback to participants and the community at large. The forum will keep the community abreast of its progress in increasing members' AIDS-related knowledge, in changing attitudes, and in reducing high-risk behaviors. These findings may also influence the changing of community norms about sexual and drug-related behaviors, such as adoption of a positive stance toward consistent condom use.

Developing Solidarity and Building Coalitions. Demands from communities of people with AIDS and communities of color have served to raise consciousness about the need for community involvement at many levels—program development, operation, and evaluation. Yet evaluations typically are developed outside the community by well-intentioned professionals. The use of what community members perceive to be an aloof approach is often implemented to ensure a stance of objectivity. However, evaluators in many policy sectors have come to accept that involvement of stakeholders, including affected communities, can improve evaluations under at least some circumstances (Mark and Shotland, 1985). Evaluators can strike a balance between community needs and scientific standards.

Involvement of community members in the design, development, implementation, and evaluation of AIDS prevention programs, including questionnaire construction, data collection, data analysis, and interpretation and dissemination of findings, must take place prior to program implementation. This involvement should maximize both the evaluators' political sensitivity to evaluation results and the effects of those results on shaping prevention policies for the targeted community. Active community involvement might also serve to defuse the anger often found in communities experiencing a disproportionate prevalence of HIV-related disease. Community reactions have ranged from mild disapproval of programs that lack a direct service component to more extreme charges of government conspiracy or ethnic genocide. Finally, community input is essential to ensure that culturally sensitive, language-appropriate prevention programs are tailored to the target group in order to minimize the chance that a program will show little or no effect. These factors underscore the importance of understanding community sensitivities when determining criteria for program impact.

Program staff, including the evaluation team, will need to network within the community to understand how to approach community leaders and institutions for program support. Community support requires that the CBO or the community itself trust the evaluator and be assured that confidentiality of information will be preserved. Obtaining community support may be accomplished best by developing a community coalition of power brokers, such as the formation of a community advisory board. The composition of such a board might include representatives from the clergy, social service and health care providers, people with HIV infection, schools, churches, businesses, politicians, and other community boards. A quarterly newsletter is another means to keep the community attuned to a program's progress.

As members feel ownership of the program, community receptivity to and acceptance of the prevention program may solidify. Without community sanction, the success of a program and its evaluation may be threatened. Securing the trust of key members of the community will provide the health educator and evaluator with access to appropriate target audiences and aid in program design and evaluation. A community support base also is an important pathway for disseminating throughout the community the importance of evaluating AIDS prevention programs.

In order to facilitate the interaction between the health educator and evaluator and the community, several formal prevention strategies and evaluation approaches can be utilized. They not only will serve to enhance community involvement but also will better shape AIDS health promotion activities to the specific needs of the community at risk.

AIDS Prevention Strategies and Evaluation Approaches

Using Social Marketing in AIDS Prevention Evaluation. Social marketing techniques have been used to improve the relevance of AIDS prevention programs, especially condom promotion, through market segmentation for populations at risk for HIV infection. It can be a useful first step in needs assessment—identifying a group's awareness of AIDS and need for preventive intervention—and it can yield important social, psychological, and behavioral information about where to target AIDS health promotion activities. Such data will also suggest strategies for reaching the audience, the messages that should be delivered, and how they should be marketed.

Social marketing evaluation allows the credibility and comprehension of messages to be assessed. For example, this approach can assess knowledge level, skills concerning correct condom usage, and resistance to adopting barrier contraception. Market analyses can also evaluate an audience's receptivity to AIDS prevention materials and channels of information diffusion. Public educational campaigns, adolescents' reactions to an AIDS rap music-video contest, and the acceptability of selling condoms in supermarkets are excellent examples.

Using Focus Groups. Formative research techniques, such as focus groups, can aid in both initial and ongoing program development where evaluation results are continuously fed back to modify the program. Focus groups have become increasingly popular in AIDS health promotion and provide another means of developing community partnerships. Focus groups entail convening a small group of people with specified characteristics in order to obtain qualitative data in a focused discussion. Methods are described in Krueger (1988).

Focus groups serve a variety of purposes in the development and evaluation of preventive interventions. In their urgency to get an AIDS prevention program up and running, education and evaluation staff may be reluctant to conduct focus groups. However, the benefits far outweigh the costs of this approach. In a relatively short period of time, focus groups can gather valuable data from relatively unstudied communities about the logistics of program implementation, program content, the appropriateness of educational materials, and the community's commitment and participation.

Logistics of Program Implementation. Focus groups and other methods of gaining community input can help determine the most efficacious means of implementing the proposed program. Appropriate recruitment and retention methods, participant incentives, number of educational sessions, best time of day for intervention, and desired characteristics of facilitators are some of the data that can be solicited from community members. In this way, provision of attractive incentives for participant enrollment and retention, such as T-shirts, money, make-up and nail grooming, self-defense lessons, child care, supportive case management, or "take-home" doses of methadone that are offered as part of a client's treatment, can be group specific (Mantell and DiVittis, in press). This approach may minimize the problems of sample size requirements and subject attrition over time and thus strengthen process and impact evaluation outcomes.

Potential barriers to program participation can be identified through these means. For example, the Gay Men's Health Crisis (GMHC) convened focus groups with black men who have sex with men (MSM) to improve their delivery of AIDS education and outreach to this population. The data revealed that GMHC's current methods of educational outreach (to large groups in community settings) were not culturally sensitive to the needs of black MSM and served as a barrier to participation. Suggested ways to provide better access to them (such as through small groups in people's homes) were outlined (Horton and Cohen, 1989).

Program Content. Input from a target group will help to develop a program formed directly by the intended audience. The New York City Department of Health's Perinatal HIV Prevention Demonstration Project is using this strategy with staff and patients to develop an educational program for women attending obstetrical and gynecological clinics (DiVittis, Jain, and Mantell, 1989). These focus groups enable the evaluator to assess patients' knowledge levels about contraception, reproductive anatomy, and HIV infection, perceptions of disease impact on friends and the community, psychological and cultural beliefs and attitudes, social norms, and the prevalence of high-risk sexual and drug-related practices; thus, priorities for topic coverage can be set.

Focus groups with MSM underscored the need for evaluators to assess perceptions of risk for HIV infection. A survey of thirty-five black and Latino MSM indicated that they had misconceptions about their personal risk of contracting AIDS. This was illustrated by such statements as "I only have sex with nice men" and "Only passive guys get AIDS" (Horton and Cohen, 1989). Such information was important to feed back into program content.

Appropriateness of Educational Materials. Both focus groups and pretesting can be used to evaluate whether the educational materials being used are appropriate for the reading level and language of the intended audience. For example, the New York City Department of Health (NYCDOH) used focus groups to develop message content for and pilot reactions to a poster placed on subways and buses and public service announcements for an AIDS prevention campaign for MSM (Vachon, 1989). In developing a new brochure about women and AIDS, the NYCDOH also conducted a series of focus groups to evaluate specific sections of the brochure with a range of women (and some men) who were infected or were at risk for HIV infection, including homeless women in shelters, seropositive women and men in a support group, women in methadone maintenance, and lesbians (Duke and others, 1989). The data collected from these groups should maximize the general appeal and appropriateness of the brochure's educational message. Groups were also conducted with service providers. Similarly, the San Francisco AIDS Foundation conducted focus groups to evaluate the messages in a newly designed condom brochure for female sex-industry workers (Spitzer, 1988).

In developing a program for recovering addicts in a residential drug-free therapeutic community, GMHC Research Program staff evaluated the appropriateness of an AIDS video that traced the history of AIDS in two individuals through their deaths. A pretest group perceived the video to be health-negative and to promote feelings of hopelessness. Based on these findings, the actual program did not use the video and averted a potential negative situation (Mantell and DiVittis, in press).

Community Commitment and Participation. Conducting focus groups with staff can provide useful information about their perceptions of the target audience and give outsiders insight into the culture of an organizational system. Engaging staff participation in the program and evaluation process may facilitate their support and thus maximize participant enrollment and program success.

Methodological Issues and Community Partnership

As in other areas of program evaluation, AIDS prevention programs are associated with a host of methodological issues. This section illustrates some of the ways in which community partnerships can help address these issues, specifically in determining definition of variables, sensitivity of evaluation instruments, criteria for program success and community-wide impact, and sampling.

Definition of Variables. Measurement problems confound our understanding of how prevention contributes to changing people's HIV risk-associated behaviors. What impact and outcome measures should be considered markers of significant behavioral change? The complexity and variations in how behavioral change is defined and made operational have made it difficult to establish meaningful evaluation measures, thus compromising the direct comparability of findings across studies.

For example, a review of major behavioral change intervention studies showed a lack of uniformity in the definition of safer-sex practice among researchers who defined the term and a lack of definition in general (Mantell and others, 1988). As study findings are disseminated to the community and shared among program staff and evaluators, it is essential that the variables under study be operationalized carefully. Both epidemiological evidence and community participation should affect this process.

Sensitivity of Evaluation Instruments. Community involvement provides a rich source for generating item pools for interview schedules or self-administered questionnaires. The appropriateness of the vernacular to describe sexual practices and literacy levels of the intended audience can be evaluated. The latter can also be accomplished by instrument pilot testing. In addition, cultural clarity of constructs and behaviors can be tested. For example, a program evaluator may learn that male homosexual behavior among Hispanics is associated with being the "receptive" sexual partner. Thus, understanding the dissonance between what people do (behavior) and how they perceive themselves or are perceived by others (social identity) may preclude the development of evaluation indicators, resulting in the underreporting of homosexual activities and, hence, erroneous conclusions about differential rates of behavioral change among blacks, Latinos, and whites. Identifying the heterogeneity among seemingly homogeneous ethnic or social groups will help to establish valid and reliable instruments.

Criteria for Program Success. Community partnerships can also help evaluators determine criteria for program success. In addition, they can be used in conjunction with epidemiological information, if it is available. For example, is reliance on statistically significant change over time sufficient to judge the success of a program aimed at eliminating HIV transmission? Typically, a statistically significant increase in condom use would represent only partial reduction in high-risk behavior (such as unprotected anal or vaginal intercourse). In cities with high HIV seroprevalence, where an estimated 50 percent of the MSM population or 60 percent of the injection drug users are infected, how successful is a program that only increases condom use? Under these circumstances, should consistent condom use or other safer-sex practices be the sole measure of success? In the absence of absolute criteria, what does the evaluator do with measures of "partial success"?

An evaluation of a four-session AIDS education program at GMHC illustrates this issue. The study revealed inconsistent condom use over time among a cohort of gay and bisexual men. By a strict criterion of consistent condom use as the only acceptable outcome, the program would have been deemed unsuccessful. However, multivariate statistical techniques enabled the evaluator to identify subsamples of the cohort for whom the intervention was effective. Through a cluster analysis, the evaluation staff identified four unique patterns of behavior in the cohort (Mantell, DiVittis, and Miller, 1989). Essentially, the clusters described men who consistently practiced safer sex at all times of assessment ("no-needs" group), men who progressed from unsafe practices to consistent safer-sex practice ("improvers"), men who went from consistent safer sex to unsafe or inconsistent safer-sex practice ("regressors"), and men who consistently practiced unsafe sex at each time of assessment ("no-change" group). Additional analyses of the characteristics of each group further identified the heterogeneity of this population. Such information can be used to tailor AIDS prevention messages to subsets of communities that previously may have been considered homogeneous.

Community Impact. The issue of behavior change has been discussed on the level of program participant. Ultimately, however, if an educational campaign is to be effective, it must be linked to community change. It must be recognized that any single intervention with a cohort drawn from a community will not result in identifiable changes in community behavior. But by carefully documenting one's efforts and the efforts of other educational campaigns and then comparing them with epidemiological trends in the community, the evaluator can link the impact of overall educational efforts with community-wide changes in behavior.

Sampling. Community partnerships have the potential to increase access to populations under study. Access should improve the representatives of the sample and the extent to which generalizations can be made about the target community. This issue becomes particularly problematic in the study of AIDS in that the size and location of the populations (for example, men who have sex with men) are often unknown. Also, the populations are difficult to reach due to the illegal nature of some risk behaviors, although some research studies have had good response rates (Hubbard and others, 1989). Further, the stigma of AIDS and the historic reliance on risk groups rather than risk behaviors have led people to deny their risk factors; for example, incarcerated men who do not identify themselves as gay or bisexual may have sex with other men. Finally, some prevention strategies (such as telephone hot lines) are designed to ensure the anonymity of their participants, making impossible representative sampling of certain target populations (such as MSM or sexual partners of injection drug users).

The few intervention studies designed for men who have sex with other men that include an evaluation component are neither population based nor drawn from random samples. Further, the inclusion criterion of "men who have sex with men" generally attracts self-identified gay men and may not speak to the larger group of men engaging in high-risk behavior with other men. For example, the use of convenience samples in programs targeted at men who have sex with men (Quadland and others, 1987; Mantell and others, 1987a, 1987b; Valdiserri and others, 1989; Joseph and others, 1987) has led to an overrepresentation of college-educated, white gay males (Mantell and others, 1989). The resultant findings are restricted to this group and not generalizable to the community at large.

Rarely does the evaluator have the luxury of true random sampling in evaluation research. In its absence, other techniques that enhance the generalizability of results are available. For example, by targeting institutions serving the population under study, such as gay clubs and organizations, the evaluator is able to recruit potential participants randomly from the ranks of the institutions (Martin and Dean, 1990). This strategy enables the evaluator to generalize findings to the membership of these institutions.

Example of Community Partnership: AIDS Hot Lines

AIDS hot lines embody many of the issues associated with evaluation of AIDS prevention programs in a community partnership. AIDS hot lines are often difficult to evaluate as most of the calls are brief and anonymous. A survey that gauges callers' perceptions of their satisfaction with the hot line (in terms of adequate referrals and appropriate support) is one means of determining both quality and effectiveness (Dozier, 1989). Measurement is limited, however, to the time immediately following a given call. To maintain anonymity, the counseling and referral needs of a caller could be handled by one hot-line worker and the subsequent evaluation of the call by another. This strategy is limiting in that impact evaluation of the hot line is restricted to knowledge and intention measures. Further, given the diverse reasons for calling, different outcomes are regulated by client need at the time of call.

Hot lines can also be evaluated from a service utilization perspective—for example, the number and length of calls, purpose of call, and, if possible, the sociodemographic background of the caller. Data bases are necessary to document this information. The evaluation will provide an assessment of the degree to which the hot line meets its stated purpose in terms of information dispersion, referrals, and a description of the people who use the service.

Another method of evaluating an AIDS education and counseling hot line is through the use of a simulation procedure (Kosecoff and Fink, 1982). This technique entails written scripts of scenarios that reflect the needs of typical hot-line callers. The people making the calls are trained in delivering the script and evaluating the performance of the hot-line counselor. The data can be used to assess the quality of the educational message, as well as the empathy and clarity of the hot-line worker's response. The technique also serves as an excellent formative evaluation measure on the effectiveness of hot-line worker training:

Conclusion

The process of program evaluation cannot exist in a vacuum. When the subject is AIDS, interaction and cooperation with the target community become essential components to successful program evaluation. The following recommendations can assist the evaluator in terms of both building relationships with the community and overcoming methodological issues in evaluation:

1. The identification of leaders and solicitation of their support will give preventive programs a stamp of approval from the target community and will engender trust from the participants.

2. Provision of continual feedback from formative and process evaluations to the community leaders in a timely manner will reinforce the partnership between the evaluation team and the community. Likewise, providing impact evaluation results to the community and participants can aid in modifying norms and facilitate community-wide adoption of risk-reduction messages.

3. Social marketing techniques assist in identifying and targeting segments of the community. Such techniques provide entrée into a community and increase awareness and acceptance of prevention messages.

4. The focus group is one formative evaluation method that can elicit qualitative data from a variety of groups in the community in a short period of time. Aside from its programmatic value, the process of participating in a focus group helps the community to invest in the project.

5. Community organizations can facilitate participant recruitment. However, generalization of results is limited by sample selection. In the absence of random sampling, the generalization of results is limited, at best, to people represented in the sample. The researchers must be cautious about overgeneralization.

6. The measurement of change in AIDS-related program evaluation requires a predetermined definition of program success that is developed in cooperation with community organizations. Further, clearly defined and culturally sensitive instruments are necessary to ensure a valid evaluation.

7. By keeping accountability to the community as the focus throughout the evaluation process, the evaluator can help ensure that the resultant findings and recommendations will have greater relevance and validity.

8. By making the community "evaluation wise," the researchers can empower community leaders to continue services beyond the funding

period. Technical assistance in grant writing, public presentation of findings, and publication of evaluation results can give something back to the community served and pave the way for future collaborative research.

9. Finally, evaluation of AIDS prevention programs enables communities to broaden the implementation of AIDS prevention initiatives that are demonstrated to be effective.

References

Archer, V. E. "Psychological Defenses and Control of AIDS." *American Journal of Public Health,* 1989, *79,* 876-878.
Braithwaite, R., and Lythcott, N. "Community Empowerment as a Strategy for Health Promotion for Black and Other Minority Populations." *Journal of the American Medical Association,* 1989, *261,* 282-283.
DiVittis, A. T., Jain, S., and Mantell, J. *Focus Group Schedule.* New York: Perinatal HIV Prevention Demonstration Project, Office of AIDS Research, New York City Department of Health, 1989.
Dozier, C. E. *AIDS Hot-Line Evaluation.* New York: Gay Men's Health Crisis, 1989.
Duke, S. I., Omi, J., Williams, R., Santiago, D., Stanley, B., Bevier, P., Porper, R., Lewis, T., Muniz, S., and Mantell, J. E. "Development of AIDS Education and Prevention Materials for Women by Health Department Staff and Community Focus Groups." Paper presented at the 117th annual meeting of the American Public Health Association, Chicago, Illinois, October 23-25, 1989.
Freudenberg, N., Lee, J., and Silver, D. "How Black and Latino Community Organizations Respond to the AIDS Epidemic: A Case Study in One New York City Neighborhood." *AIDS Education and Prevention,* 1989, *1,* 12-21.
Horton, R., and Cohen, M. *A Survey of AIDS Knowledge, Attitudes, and Behaviors of Men of Color Who Have Sex with Men and Reactions to the Leaflet "Brothers Loving Brothers Safely": Summary of Results.* New York: Gay Men's Health Crisis, 1989.
Hubbard, R. L., Marsden, M. E., Rachal, J. V., Harwood, H. J., Cavanaugh, E. R., and Ginzburg, H. M. *Drug Abuse Treatment.* Chapel Hill: University of North Carolina Press, 1989.
Joseph, J., Montgomery, S., Emmons, C., Kessler, R. C., Ostrow, D. G., Wortman, C. B., O'Brien, K., Eller, M., and Eshleman, S. "Magnitude and Determinants of Behavioral Risk Reduction: Longitudinal Analysis of a Cohort at Risk for AIDS." *Psychology and Health,* 1987, *1,* 73-96.
Judson, F. "What Do We Really Know About AIDS Control?" *American Journal of Public Health,* 1989, *79,* 878-882.
Kosecoff, J., and Fink, A. *Evaluation Basics—A Practitioner's Manual.* Newbury Park, Calif.: Sage, 1982.
Krueger, R. *Focus Groups: A Practical Guide for Applied Research.* Newbury Park, Calif.: Sage, 1988.
Mantell, J. E., and DiVittis, A. T. *Evaluating AIDS Prevention Programs: A Guidebook for the Health Educator.* New York: Gay Men's Health Crisis, in press.
Mantell, J. E., DiVittis, A. T., and Miller, R. *The STUDY—Final Report Submitted to the Centers for Disease Control for Gay Men's Health Crisis.* New York: Gay Men's Health Crisis, 1989.
Mantell, J. E., DiVittis, A. T., Spivak, H., Kochems, L., Simon, S., Mahony, K., Ostfield, M. L., Holmes, J., Winters, D., Eisen, K., and Patruch, C. "A Meta-Analysis

of AIDS Behavioral Research: Methodological and Political Issues." Presentation made at the Fourth International Conference on AIDS, Stockholm, Sweden, June 12-16, 1988.

Mantell, J. E., DiVittis, A. T., Whittier, D., Shifflet, S., and Ahuja, H. "AIDS Health Promotion Among Males Who Have Sex with Males in New York City." Paper presented at the World Health Organization's Global Program on AIDS, Workshop on AIDS Health Promotional Activities Directed Toward Gay and Bisexual Men, Geneva, Switzerland, May 1989.

Mantell, J. E., Kochems, L., DiVittis, A. T., Mahony, K., Mastroianni, P., McKinney, C., Blaustein, D., and Ketcham, M. "An Erotic/Nonpornographic Video Educational Program for AIDS Risk Reduction for Gay and Bisexual Men." Presentation made at the National Lesbian and Gay Health Conference/Fifth National AIDS Forum. Los Angeles, California, March 1987a.

Mantell, J. E., Kochems, L., DiVittis, A. T., Mastroianni, P., Mahony, K., McKinney, C., Ketcham, M., and Blaustein, D. "A Randomized Community-Based Risk Reduction Educational Intervention for Gay and Bisexual Men." Paper presented at the National Lesbian and Gay Health Conference/Fifth National AIDS Forum. Los Angeles, California, March 1987b.

Mark, M. M., and Shotland, R. L. "Stakeholder-Based Evaluation and Value Judgments." *Evaluation Review*, 1985, 9 (5), 605-625.

Martin, J. L., and Dean, L. "Developing a Community Sample of Gay Men for an Epidemiologic Study of AIDS." *American Behavioral Scientist*, 1990, 33, 546-561.

Potterat, J. J., Spencer, N. E., Woodhouse, D. E., and Muth, J. B. "Partner Notification in the Control of Human Immunodeficiency Virus Infection." *American Journal of Public Health*, 1989, 79, 874-876.

Quadland, M. C., Schuman, R., Shattls, W., Jacobs, R., and D'Eramo, J. "The 800 Men Study." Paper presented at the First International Lesbian and Gay Health Conference and AIDS Forum, Los Angeles, July 1987.

Spitzer, S. *Focus Group Report: Condom Distribution Piece.* San Francisco: San Francisco AIDS Foundation, 1988.

Vachon, R. Personal communication. June 1989.

Valdiserri, R. O., Lyter, D. W., Leviton, L. C., Callahan, C. M., Kingsley, L. A., and Rinaldo, C. R. "AIDS Prevention in Homosexual and Bisexual Men: Results of a Randomized Trial Evaluating Two Risk-Reduction Interventions." *AIDS*, 1989, 3, 21-26.

Joanne E. Mantell is senior research scientist at the Office of AIDS Research, New York City Department of Health, and principal investigator of a knowledge-attitude-behavior survey of women receiving obstetrical and gynecological services and of a perinatal HIV prevention demonstration project.

Anthony T. DiVittis is currently finishing his doctoral work in psychometrics at Fordham University in New York and is working on a perinatal HIV risk-reduction project with the New York City Department of Health, AIDS Research Unit.

Name Index

Abramson, P. R., 3, 28, 30, 34, 37, 47, 49
Adler, N. E., 8, 21
Ahuja, H., 98
Ajzen, I., 76, 84
Allain, J.-P., 84
Amemiya, T., 41, 45, 46, 47
Ancelle, R. A., 35
Anderson, R. E., 22
Anderson, R. M., 25, 26, 27, 28, 29, 30, 34, 36, 38, 40, 42, 47, 49
Antoniskis, D., 52, 61
Archer, V. E., 88, 97
Atkin, C. K., 67, 71

Bacchetti, P., 25, 35
Bailey, N.T.J., 37, 47
Bandura, A., 14, 19, 20
Barger, K., 54, 61
Barnett, V., 45, 47
Barraj, L. M., 40, 47, 48
Baum, A., 9, 20
Becker, M. H., 9, 18, 20, 21, 53, 61, 75, 76, 83, 84
Bell, N. K., 2, 6
Benfari, R. C., 70, 71
Berk, R. A., 3, 37, 41, 45, 46, 47, 49
Bernard, H. R., 54, 55, 61
Bevier, P., 97
Billard, L., 25, 28, 30, 36, 38, 49
Blanchard, J., 9, 20
Blaustein, D., 98
Blower, S. M., 29, 36, 40, 42, 49
Blum, M. R., 84
Boccellari, A., 84
Boruch, R., 19, 21
Bowen, G. S., 61
Boyer, C. B., 52, 61
Braithwaite, R., 88, 97
Brandt, E. N., 34, 35
Bregman, D. J., 48
Broder, S., 84
Brookmeyer, R., 25, 35, 47
Brown, B., 2, 6
Brunet, J. B., 35
Bryer, S., 75, 85

Callahan, C. M., 21, 22, 98
Cameron, D. W., 49

Carleton, R. A., 20
Caroni, C., 26, 36
Catania, J. A., 9, 15, 20
Cavanaugh, E. F., 97
Chin, J., 49
Chmiel, J., 21, 48
Clark, L., 75, 85
Coates, T. J., 9, 15, 20, 64, 69, 70, 72, 75, 84
Cochran, S. D., 68, 72
Cohen, F., 8, 21
Cohen, M., 91, 92, 97
Cohen, R., 62
Conant, M., 64, 69, 70, 72
Conner, R. F., 4, 75, 85
Cook, T. D., 2, 6
Corby, N., 9, 20
Cox, C., 62
Cox, D. R., 25, 28, 30, 36, 38, 49
Coyle, S., 19, 21
Cramton, P. C., 28, 34, 35
Curran, J. W., 24, 25, 35, 39, 40, 47, 49, 63, 72

Dalgorn, R., 52, 61
Dans, P. E., 75, 84
Darrow, W. W., 20, 25, 28, 30, 36
Davis, D. L., 13, 21
D'Costa, L. J., 48
De Gruttola, V., 40, 47, 48
Dean, L., 95, 98
DeBoor, M., 52, 61
DeHovitz, J. A., 39, 48
Dennis, M., 5
D'Eramo, J., 72, 98
Des Jarlais, D. C., 9, 20, 66, 72
Detels, R., 48
Detre, K., 48
DeVellis, B. M., 8, 21
DeVellis, R. F., 8, 21
Devine, O. J., 24, 36
DiClemente, R. J., 52, 61
Dietz, K., 29, 35, 47, 48
DiVittis, A. T., 1, 5, 87, 91, 92, 94, 97, 98
Doll, L. S., 9, 20
Dondero, T. J., 47
Dougherty, J., 63, 72

Downing, M., 51, 61
Downs, A. M., 24, 35
Dozier, C. E., 95, 97
Drotman, D. P., 61
Duke, S. I., 92, 97
Dunbar, J., 5

Edwards, M., 5
Eisen, K., 98
Elder, J. R., 8, 9, 20
Elkers, J., 13, 21
Eller, M., 21, 97
Ellickson, P. L., 69, 72
Emmons, C., 97
Eraker, S. A., 76, 84
Eshleman, S., 97
Essex, M., 39, 48
Estrada, A. L., 52, 61
Evans, A. S., 37, 48

Fagan, R., 9, 21
Fan, H., 75
Farquhar, J. W., 76, 84
Fauci, A. S., 49
Feiner, C., 62
Feinsod, F. M., 49
Feldblum, P. J., 53, 61
Feldman, D. A., 51, 61
Fernandez, M., 52, 61
Fetterman, D., 54, 60, 61
Fineberg, H. V., 53, 61, 64, 72, 75, 84
Fink, A., 95, 97
Fischl, M. A., 53, 61
Fishbein, M., 76, 84
Flam, R., 52, 61
Fortney, J. A., 53, 61
Francis, D. P., 39, 48
Franzini, L., 8, 9, 21
Freeman, H., 37
Freeman, H. E., 2, 6, 55, 62
Freudenberg, N., 5, 6, 88, 97
Friedman, S. R., 9, 20, 66, 72

Gail, M. H., 25, 30-31, 35, 47
Galavotti, C., 8, 9, 20, 21
Gallion, K. J., 8, 9, 20
Gibson, D. R., 20
Gilmore, N., 75, 84
Ginsburg, H. M., 97
Glaser, K., 9, 20
Glunt, E. K., 9, 20
Goetz, J., 54, 61

Goldberger, A. S., 44, 45, 46, 48
Grant, R., 22, 29, 30, 35
Greenblatt, R. M., 20
Grell, L. S., 54, 62
Guttman, M., 4, 6

Hadeler, K. P., 47, 48
Hahn, R. A., 63, 72
Hardy, A. M., 47, 63, 72
Harwood, H. J., 97
Haverkos, H. W., 48
Heckman, J. J., 46, 48
Hegedus, A. M., 5, 6
Hein, K., 63, 66, 72
Heisterkamp, S. H., 24, 35
Herek, G. M., 9, 20
Herschkorn, S. J., 29, 36
Hessol, N., 20
Heyward, W. L., 24, 25, 35
Hirsch, D. A., 9, 21
Ho, D. D., 37, 48
Hochbaum, G. M., 8, 21
Hoff, C. C., 64, 72
Holland, P. W., 46, 47, 48
Holmes, J., 98
Holmes, K. K., 48
Hood, J. S., 68, 69, 72
Hopkins, D. R., 52, 61
Horton, R., 91, 92, 97
Hovell, M., 8, 9, 20, 21
Hubbard, R. L., 94, 97
Hull, F., 75, 84
Hurtado, E., 60, 62
Hyman, J. M., 25, 28, 29, 35

Isham, V., 47, 48

Jackonia, O. N., 49
Jacobs, R., 72, 98
Jacobsen, F. K., 84
Jacquez, J., 28, 35, 36
Jaffe, H. W., 47, 63, 72
Jager, J. C., 35
Jain, S., 91, 97
Janz, N. K., 76, 84
Jimerez, J., 75
Johnson, A. M., 26, 27, 28, 34
Johnson, T. M., 51, 61
Jones, T. S., 63, 72
Joseph, J., 21, 36, 64, 72, 95, 97
Joseph, J. G., 9, 20, 53, 61, 75, 84
Judson, F., 88, 97

Name Index

Kahan, J. P., 69, 72
Kalsey, S. F., 48
Kapita, B., 49
Kaplan, E. H., 3, 5, 23, 26, 27, 28, 29, 30, 31–32, 34, 35, 36, 38, 39, 48
Kaplan, J. C., 37, 47, 48
Karon, J. M., 24, 36
Kaslow, R., 48
Kegeles, S. M., 15, 20
Kelly, J. A., 9, 15, 19, 20, 68, 69, 72
Kelsey, J. L., 37, 48
Kendall, O., 75, 84
Kessler, H. A., 84
Kessler, R., 21
Kessler, R. C., 97
Ketcham, M., 98
Kiecolt-Glaser, J. K., 9, 20
Kincade, R. L., 9, 20
Kingsley, L. A., 21, 22, 39, 48, 98
Kinosian, B. P., 75, 84
Kirscht, J. P., 76, 84
Kleiman, M.A.R., 32, 36
Klein, R., 75, 84
Kochems, L., 98
Koech, D., 48
Kolbe, L., 61
Koopman, J., 28, 35, 36
Kosecoff, J., 95, 97
Kreiss, J. D., 49
Kreiss, J. K., 39, 48
Krueger, R., 91, 97
Kubrin, A., 5, 6

Lagakos, S. W., 40, 47, 48
Lai, M., 75, 85
Lamboray, J., 49
Lang, W., 22
Lasater, T. M., 20
Lawless, J. F., 40, 42, 45, 46, 48
Lawrence, D. N., 48
LeCompte, M., 54, 61
Lee, J., 5, 6, 88, 97
Leedom, J. M., 52, 61
Lehrman, S. N., 84
Leuther, M., 84
Leventhal, H., 4, 6
Leviton, L. C., 2, 5, 6, 9, 15, 20, 21, 22, 84, 98
Levy, J. A., 22, 39, 40, 48
Lewis, M. A., 75, 85
Lewis, T., 97
Lieb, L. E., 36

Lifson, A., 20
Lightfoote, M., 48
Lindsey, B., 61
Lipshutz, C., 62
Little, R.J.A., 37
Longshore, D., 4, 63, 73
Lui, K., 38, 48
Lui, K.-J., 25, 28, 30, 36, 38, 39, 48
Lyman, D. M., 22
Lyter, D. W., 21, 22, 84, 98
Lythcott, N., 88, 97

McAlister, A., 8, 9, 20
McAtee, N., 84
Maccoby, N., 67, 72
McCormick, J. B., 49
McGuire, W. J., 67, 68, 72
McIntyre, K. M., 70, 71
McKinney, C., 98
McKusick, L., 9, 20, 64, 69, 70, 72, 84
Maha, M., 84
Mahony, K., 98
Maiman, L. A., 76, 84
Mandel, J. S., 9, 21, 84
Manderscheid, R. W., 13, 21
Mann, J. M., 39, 40, 49
Manski, C. F., 47, 48
Mantell, J., 1, 5, 87, 91, 92, 94, 95, 97, 98
Marin, B., 20
Mark, M. M., 89, 98
Marks, J., 75, 85
Marlik, R. G., 39, 48
Marsden, M. E., 97
Martin, J., 9, 20, 95, 98
Mason, J. O., 52, 61
Mastroianni, P., 98
May, R. M., 26, 27, 28, 29, 30, 34, 36, 38, 40, 42, 47, 49
Mays, V. M., 68, 72
Medley, G. F., 25, 26, 27, 28, 30, 34, 36, 38, 49
Meyer, D., 4, 6
Mhalu, F. S., 49
Miller, H. G., 19, 21
Miller, R., 94, 97
Mishra, S. I., 75, 85
Mitsuya, H., 84
Mockler, R. A., 32, 36
Mondanaro, J., 2, 6
Montgomery, S., 97
Morales, E. F., 84

Morales, E. S., 52, 61
Morgan, W. M., 24, 36, 47, 48
Morin, G., 9, 21
Morin, S., 9, 15, 20, 21, 84
Moses, L. E., 19, 21
Moss, A. R., 25, 35
Moulton, J. M., 9, 21
Muniz, S., 97
Muth, J. B., 88, 98
Myers, C. E., 84

Ndinya-achola, J. O., 48
Nesselhof, S.E.A., 9, 20
Newmeyer, J., 70, 72
Ng, L.K.Y., 13, 21
Ngugi, E. N., 48, 49
Noble, G., 61

O'Brien, K., 97
Ockene, J. K., 70, 71
Odaka, N., 48
O'Malley, P., 20
Omi, J., 97
Onorato, I. M., 63, 72
O'Reilly, K. R., 9, 21
Ostfield, M. L., 98
Ostrow, D., 13, 15, 21, 48, 97

Padian, N., 22
Padian, N. S., 29, 36
Page, J. B., 51, 62
Paltiel, A. D., 28, 34, 35
Papaevangelou, G., 26, 36
Park, T., 36
Parry, T., 35
Pascal, A., 1, 6
Patruch, C., 98
Pelto, G. H., 54, 55, 62
Pelto, P. J., 54, 55, 62
Pershing, A., 20
Peterman, T. A., 48
Peterson, J. L., 9, 21, 52, 62
Phair, J., 21
Piantadosi, S., 30-31, 35
Pickering, J., 26, 36
Piot, P., 38, 39, 40, 42, 48, 49
Pluda, J. M., 84
Plummer, F. A., 48, 49
Polich, J. M., 69, 72
Polk, B. F., 48
Pomerantz, R. J., 37, 47, 48
Porper, R., 97

Potterat, J. J., 88, 98
Preston, D., 30-31, 35
Prue, D. M., 14, 21

Quadland, M. C., 69, 72, 95, 98
Quinn, T. C., 39, 40, 48, 49

Rachal, J. V., 97
Ramirez, A. G., 8, 9, 20
Resnicow, K. A., 14, 21
Reuter, P., 69, 72
Reza, E., 54, 61
Rhodes, F., 9, 20, 78, 84
Richards, M., 75
Richardson, S. C., 26, 36
Richwald, G. A., 53, 62
Riggs, J., 22
Rinaldo, C. R., 21, 22, 48, 98
Roberts, D. F., 67, 72
Roberts, P., 48
Romney, A. K., 54, 62
Ronald, A. R., 48
Rosenberg, M., 61
Rosenstock, I. M., 18, 21, 76, 84
Rossi, P. H., 2, 6, 55, 62
Rothschild, B., 28, 34, 47
Rubin, D. B., 46, 48
Rugg, D., 3, 4, 7, 8, 9, 21, 22
Ruitenberg, E. J., 35
Runyan, C. W., 8, 21
Rutherford, G. W., III, 25, 28, 30, 36, 38, 39, 48

St. Lawrence, J. S., 9, 15, 19, 20, 68, 69, 72
Sallis, J. F., 9, 20
Samuel, M., 22
Santiago, D., 97
Sartwell, P. E., 37, 49
Sattenspiel, L., 35, 36
Sattler, F. R., 52, 61
Scharf, L. S., 14, 21
Schensul, J. J., 3, 51, 54, 62
Schensul, S. L., 3, 51, 54, 62
Schneider, H., 41, 46, 49
Schneider-Monoz, M., 53, 62
Schoepfle, G. M., 54, 62
Schott, J. R., 68, 70, 72
Schulberg, H., 5
Schuman, R., 72, 98
Schwartz, J., 75, 84
Scrimshaw, S.C.M., 60, 62
Sechrest, L., 3, 6

Name Index

Selik, R. M., 47
Selwyn, P. A., 53, 62
Sevilla-Casa, E., 54, 62
Shadish, W. R., 2, 5, 6
Shattls, W., 72, 98
Shifflet, S., 98
Shilts, R., 1, 6
Shotland, R. L., 89, 98
Silver, D., 5, 6, 88, 97
Silverman, M., 5
Silvestre, A., 84
Simon, C. P., 35, 36
Simon, S., 98
Simoneson, J. N., 49
Sorensen, J. L., 84
Sotheran, J. L., 66, 72
Soucey, J., 21
Spencer, N. E., 88, 98
Spitzer, S., 92, 98
Spivak, H., 98
Stall, R., 9, 20, 64, 72, 84
Stanley, B., 97
Stanley, E. A., 25, 28, 29, 35
Stein, Z., 52, 61
Sterk, C., 51, 62
Stevens, W., 49
Stone, G. C., 8, 21
Stoner, K., 84
Strecher, V. J., 18, 21, 76, 84
Stull, D., 54, 62
Suchman, E., 55, 62
Surbone, A., 75, 84
Sutton, S. R., 68, 71, 73
Sweet, D. M., 9, 21

Taelman, H., 49
Taylor, J.M.G., 26, 36
Taylor, S. E., 8, 21
Temoshok, L., 9, 21, 22
Thomas, R. V., 84
Thompson, W. D., 37, 48

Tross, S., 9, 21
Turner, C. F., 19, 21

Vachon, R., 92, 98
Valdez, R. B., 53, 62
Valdiserri, R. O., 2, 6, 9, 13, 19, 20, 21, 22, 75, 84, 95, 98
van Druten, J.A.M., 35
Van Ness, 61
VanRaden, M., 48
Villareal, L., 75
Visscher, B., 48

Wainberg, M. A., 75, 84
Walker, J., 36
Wallston, B. S., 76, 84
Wallston, K. A., 76, 84
Weinstein, N. D., 77, 84
Weller, S. C., 54, 62
Wells, B. L., 20
Werner, O., 54, 62
Weston, T., 54, 62
Whittier, D., 98
Wiebel, W. W., 4, 6
Wiley, J., 22, 29, 30, 35, 36, 84
Williams, L. S., 66, 67, 73
Williams, R., 97
Winkelstein, W., 18, 22, 29, 30, 35
Winters, D., 98
Wolcott, H., 55, 62
Wolitski, R. J., 9, 20, 78, 84
Woodhouse, D. E., 88, 98
Wortman, C. B., 97
Wynder, E. L., 14, 21

Yarchoan, R., 84
Yeaton, W. H., 3, 6

Zich, J., 9, 22

Subject Index

AIDS: models for forecasting, 24-26; number of cases of, 1, 23; stages of, 11-12
AIDS Community Research Group, 52, 61
AIDS education: class for, 77-83; impact continuum for, 12-15; materials for, 92; model campaigns of, 64-65; model for, 65-70; and other public health issues, 70-71
AIDS Fundamentals class, 77-83
AIDS hot lines, 95-96
AIDS incubation periods, 37-38, 47; external validity of, with convenience samples, 38-41; internal validity of, with convenience samples, 41-47
AIDS prevention: class for, 77-83; and community, 94-95; and methodological issues, 92-94; model campaigns for, 64-65; multilevel framework for, 9-11; and public health psychology, 9; public health psychology concepts in, 9-18; strategies for, 90-92

Bayview-Hunter's Point Foundation, 65, 69
Behavior: adverse, 32-33; change of, after class, 81, 82; continuums for, 12, 15-18; ethnography and AIDS-related, 53-55; and health psychology, 8; high-risk, 2; skills for changing, 68; theories on health-related, 4, 76-77
Behavior-Change Continuum, 15-18

Campaigns, model AIDS prevention, 64-65. *See also* AIDS education; Programs
Censoring, 40, 41-46
Center for New Schools, 54, 61
Centers for Disease Control (CDC), 1, 6, 11, 12, 20, 23, 24, 35, 64, 72
Community: and AIDS hot lines, 95-96; and AIDS prevention, 94-95
Community-based organizations (CBOs), 87; and evaluation, 88-90
Continuum: Behavior-Change, 15-18; of Impact Potential for AIDS Education Strategies, 12-14; Relative-Risk Behavioral, 12
Drug use. *See* Injection drug users (IDUs); Intravenous drug users

Education, AIDS. *See* AIDS education
Ethnographic evaluation, 55-56; steps in, 56-59
Ethnographic research, on AIDS-related behavior, 53-55
Ethnography, 51-52, 60
Evaluation: of AIDS prevention, 1-2; approaches for, 90-92; collaborative, 88-89; and community, 96-97; ethnographic, 55-59; recommendations for, 18-19; theory-based, 75-83

Focus groups, 90-92
Forecasting, mathematical models for, 24-26

GAO. *See* U.S. General Accounting Office (GAO)
Gay Men's Health Crisis (GMHC), 5, 91, 92, 94

Health Belief Model (HBM), 76
Health Decision Model (HDM), 76-77
Health psychology, 8
Health Watch, 65, 68
Hispanic Health Alliance, 52, 61
HIV screening, mathematical model for, 30-31
HIV transmission, 12; and adverse behavior, 32-33; mathematical models of, 26-29, 31
Hot lines. *See* AIDS hot lines

Incubation, 37. *See also* AIDS incubation periods
Injection drug users (IDUs), 2, 4; and Behavioral Change Continuum, 15-17; collecting information on, 59; and ethnographic evaluation, 51, 56-57, 58, 59; model for HIV transmission by, 31; and Relative-Risk Behavioral Continuum, 12. *See also* Intravenous drug users
Institute for Community Research, 55, 61
Intravenous drug users, as target group, 63, 65. *See also* Injection drug users (IDUs)

Los Alamos National Laboratory, 24

Los Angeles, 64; model AIDS prevention campaigns in, 65

Mathematical model(s), 23, 34; and adverse behavior, 32-33; for forecasting, 24-26; for HIV transmission dynamics, 26-29; for policies, 29-32
Media, and AIDS prevention campaigns, 67
Minorities, 66-67; as target group, 63, 65
Model(s): Health Belief, 76; Health Decision, 76-77; mathematical, 23-32, 34; Precaution-Adoption Process, 77. See also Continuum
Motivators, in AIDS prevention campaigns, 68-69

National Organizations Responding to AIDS, 1, 6
New York City, 64; model AIDS prevention campaigns in, 65
New York City Department of Health, 5, 91, 92

Office of Technology Assessment, 63, 72

Policy, mathematical models of, 29-32
Precaution-Adoption Process Model (PAP), 77
Prevention. See AIDS prevention
Programs: community and AIDS prevention, 87-97; ethnographic evaluation of, 56-59. See also Campaigns

Project COPE, 59
Project Return, 65, 68
Psychology: health, 8; public health, 8-9
Public health, AIDS and other issues for, 70-71
Public health psychology, 8-9; and AIDS prevention, 9-18

Relative-Risk Behavioral Continuum, 12
Research: ethnographic, 53-55; gaps in AIDS-related, 52-53

Safer sex, mathematical model for, 30
San Francisco, 64; model AIDS prevention campaigns in, 65
San Francisco AIDS Foundation, 65, 68, 92
Skills, for changing behavior, 68
Social marketing, in AIDS prevention evaluation, 90

Target groups, 63; for education, 66; for prevention campaigns, 65
Truncation, 41

U.S. General Accounting Office (GAO), 4, 67, 69, 70, 73; AIDS education model of, 63-70

Vaccine, mathematical model for immunizing, 31-32

World Health Organization, 39, 40, 49

Youth, as target group, 63, 65

ORDERING INFORMATION

NEW DIRECTIONS FOR PROGRAM EVALUATION is a series of paperback books that presents the latest techniques and procedures for conducting useful evaluation studies of all types of programs. Books in the series are published quarterly in Fall, Winter, Spring, and Summer and are available for purchase by subscription as well as by single copy.

SUBSCRIPTIONS for 1990 cost $48.00 for individuals (a savings of 20 percent over single-copy prices) and $64.00 for institutions, agencies, and libraries. Please do not send institutional checks for personal subscriptions. Standing orders are accepted.

SINGLE COPIES cost $14.95 when payment accompanies order. (California, New Jersey, New York, and Washington, D.C., residents please include appropriate sales tax.) Billed orders will be charged postage and handling.

DISCOUNTS FOR QUANTITY ORDERS are available. Please write to the address below for information.

ALL ORDERS must include either the name of an individual or an official purchase order number. Please submit your order as follows:
  Subscriptions: specify series and year subscription is to begin
  Single copies: include individual title code (such as PE1)

MAIL ALL ORDERS TO:
  Jossey-Bass Inc., Publishers
  350 Sansome Street
  San Francisco, California 94104

OTHER TITLES AVAILABLE IN THE
NEW DIRECTIONS FOR PROGRAM EVALUATION SERIES
Nick L. Smith, *Editor-in-Chief*

PE45 Evaluation and Social Justice: Issues in Public Education, *Kenneth A. Sirotnik*
PE44 Evaluating Training Programs in Business and Industry,
 Robert O. Brinkerhoff
PE43 Evaluating Health Promotion Programs, *Marc T. Braverman*
PE42 International Innovations in Evaluation Methodology, *Ross F. Conner,
 Michael Hendricks*
PE41 Evaluation and the Federal Decision Maker, *Gerald L. Barkdoll,
 James B. Bell*
PE40 Evaluating Program Environments, *Kendon J. Conrad,
 Cynthia Roberts-Gray*
PE39 Evaluation Utilization, *John A. McLaughlin, Larry J. Weber,
 Robert W. Covert, Robert B. Ingle*
PE38 Timely, Lost-Cost Evaluation in the Public Sector, *Christopher G. Wye,
 Harry P. Hatry*
PE37 Lessons from Selected Program and Policy Areas, *Howard S. Bloom,
 David S. Cordray, Richard J. Light*
PE36 The Client Perspective on Evaluation, *Jeri Nowakowski*
PE35 Multiple Methods in Program Evaluation, *Melvin M. Mark,
 R. Lance Shotland*
PE34 Evaluation Practice in Review, *David S. Cordray, Howard S. Bloom,
 Richard J. Light*
PE33 Using Program Theory in Evaluation, *Leonard Bickman*
PE32 Measuring Efficiency: An Assessment of Data Envelopment Analysis,
 Richard H. Silkman
PE31 Advances in Quasi-Experimental Design and Analysis,
 William M. K. Trochim
PE30 Naturalistic Evaluation, *David D. Williams*
PE29 Teaching of Evaluation Across the Disciplines, *Barbara Gross Davis*
PE28 Randomization and Field Experimentation, *Robert F. Boruch,
 Werner Wothke*
PE27 Utilizing Prior Research in Evaluation Planning, *David S. Cordray*
PE26 Economic Evaluations of Public Programs, *James S. Catterall*